HEALTH CAPITAL FINANCING

HEALTH CAPITAL FINANCING

Structuring Politics and Markets to Produce Community Health

Jonathan Betz Brown

with Stephen R. Thomas and members of the Harvard University Health Capital Project

Health Administration Press Perspectives
Ann Arbor, Michigan
1988

Library of Congress Cataloging-in-Publication Data

Brown, Jonathan Betz.
Health capital financing: structuring politics and markets to produce community health / Jonathan Betz Brown with Stephen R. Thomas and members of the Harvard University Health Capital Project.
p. cm.
Includes index.
ISBN 0-910701-27-X
1. Harvard University. Health Capital Project. 2. Health facilities—Design and construction—Finance. 3. Capital investments. 4. Health facilities—United States—Planning—History. I. Thomas, Stephen R. (Stephen Richard), 1943–
II. Harvard University. Health Capital Project. III. Title.
[DNLM: 1. Community Health Services—economics—United States. 2. Financial Management—economics—United States. 3. Health Planning—economics—United States. 4. Health Policy—trends—United States. WA 546 AA1 B82h]
RA967.B83 1987 362.1'068'1—dc19
DNLM/DLC for Library of Congress 87-34226 CIP

Health Administration Press
A Division of the Foundation of the
American College of Healthcare Executives
1021 East Huron Street
Ann Arbor, Michigan 48104-9990
(313) 764-1380

For
C. Rufus Rorem, Ph.D.,
author of the first (and still one of the best) books about health capital in the United States and a long-standing proponent of community management of health resources
and
Robert M. Sigmond,
Rorem's student, a leader in the voluntary health planning movement of the 1960s and an articulate advocate of capital pooling and community governance, who gave generously of his time and experience to help improve this book

TABLE OF CONTENTS

LIST OF EXHIBITS

ACKNOWLEDGMENTS

This book taught me to distinguish two kinds of academic collaboration. The first kind—and it is a valuable kind—might be termed "potluck collaboration." Each participant brings a dish basically of his or her own making, and the project leader soon learns, or already knows, that each will use a recipe not much different from the one he or she used for the last project.[1] There can be a certain kind of efficiency in this division of labor but, as Benjamin Barber remarks of the view that the sole responsibility of business is to increase its profits, "The problem . . . is not that it asks men to be greedy or competitive but that it asks them to be *unimaginative*."[2]

"Design collaboration" demands a good deal more imagination. It requires a good deal more work, as well. The participants must commit themselves to take seriously and to solve—not just analyze or comment on—a specific problem. They must take the time to reach a common understanding of its causes and agree on why it deserves a solution. They must spend considerable time creating, communicating, and mutually criticizing ideas about how to solve it, especially if it is a new and difficult sort of problem. If the problem also is a large one that requires a division of labor, each participant must additionally accept that the solution to his part or her part depends on how fellow collaborators solve the other parts. This interdependency makes it tough on authors of the downstream chapters when the hoped-for solution must be communicated in the linear, concatenated form of a book.

Many individuals and institutions contributed to the writing of this book. First and foremost, I take pleasure in thanking my principal coauthor, Stephen R. Thomas, for his stimulating intellectual and human companionship throughout the endeavor and for his whole-hearted willingness to join forces in the uncertain task of institutional design. Steve's knowledge and love for political theory and public management helped the book grow beyond the narrow confines of health policy tinkering. His Chapter 5 holds insights for a broad range of political theorists and policy leaders.

I also take pleasure in acknowledging the contributions of David W. Young, now Professor of Accounting and Control in the Boston University School of Management. David's knowledge of capital planning in other industries provided an instructive model for community capital allocation in health care, as did the case study of the Massachusetts Housing Finance Agency that he wrote with Lynn Jenkins. This case study appears in the present volume as Appendix B. A neighbor as well as a colleague, I thank David most sincerely for his friendship and his contributions to the book.

In addition to being coauthor of Appendix B, Lynn Jenkins served the Health Capital Project as its principal research staff person for more than two years. All who participated in the project are indebted to Lynn for her commitment as well as her competence.

Several other faculty members formerly or currently in the Department of Health Policy and Management at the Harvard School of Public Health contributed to the Health Capital Project and to the discourse that led ultimately to this book. Richard B. Saltman and I coauthored an article that subsequently appeared in *Inquiry* ("Health Capital Policy in the United States: A Strategic Perspective," 22 [Summer 1985]: 122–31) in which early forms of some of the ideas that appear in early chapters of the book were first set down. I would like particularly to thank Penny Hollander Feldman, Nancy M. Kane, Marc J. Roberts, and Richard B. Saltman. Other individuals, from Harvard and elsewhere, participated actively in Health Capital Project seminars and working groups or provided useful advice at crucial moments. These include Peter Buck, Phillip Caper, Donald Cohodes, Barry Ensminger, Rashi Fein, Harvey Fineberg, William Hsiao, John Iglehart, David Kinzer, Mitchell Rabkin, Ginger Makay-Smith, Harry M. Marks, Frederick Mosteller, Katherine Pell, Julius Richmond, and Pedro Saturno.

Regina Anderson served ably as secretary to the Health Capital Project throughout its life, typing manuscripts, maintaining the bibliographic retrieval system, and trying to keep everyone organized. She was competently and compassionately supported by Deborah Harris, who managed the clerical and technical resources in the Department of Health Policy and Management; by Theresa Campos and Lisa Fauteaux, who kept the books; and by other members of the secretarial staff including Judith Arsenault and Jenny Taylor, who may someday write an academic book of her own. Shana Levy helped get the book over the final hump and into the publisher's hands in reasonable shape.

The Josiah Macy, Jr. Foundation of New York City supported financially the preparation of this book and served as lead funding agency for the Health Capital Project which spawned it. Maxine Bleich, now Vice President of the Foundation, was a supportive overseer throughout the project. My colleagues and I are most grateful to the Macy Foundation and to Maxine. The Equitable Life Assurance Society of America, Inc. and its Vice President, Arthur Lifson, joined the Macy Foundation to support the book. Other funders of an earlier phase of the Health Capital Project included the Charitable Foundation of the Morgan Guaranty Trust Company of New York City, Inc., the New York Community Trust, Inc., and the United Hospital Fund of New York City.

Throughout the project, I benefited from the supervisory as well as the intellectual support of two Harvard luminaries. Dr. Julius Richmond, who led Harvard's universitywide Division of Health Care Policy Research and Education during the course of the project, provided vital impetus in getting the Health Capital Project off the ground and keeping it aloft. Frederick Mosteller, a true polymath and renowned master organizer of academic collaboration, taught me much about project leadership, some of which I was smart enough to use. Dr. Mosteller led the Department of Health Policy and Management in the Harvard School of Public Health.

On behalf of Steve Thomas, I would like to thank the health policy leaders in Rochester, New York, who so generously gave him access to their files and experience as he prepared his case study of capital pooling in the Hospital Experimental Payments Program: Richard Berman, Sarah Hartmann, Claire Lovinski, Donna Regenstreif, and Michael Weidner. On David Young's behalf, I thank the leaders and constituents of the Massachusetts Housing Finance Agency who were equally helpful and supportive.

This book is a better book than it would otherwise be thanks to the thoughtful and professional editors at Health Administration Press, Gene Regenstreif and Daphne Grew. Nancy J. Moncrieff edited the text with exacting insight that went well beyond her mastery of grammar and style: she sometimes knew more about the topic than any of the authors.

I dedicate the book to Robert Sigmond, who has been thinking, writing, and speaking about many of the same ideas for decades, and to his mentor, C. Rufus Rorem, one of the towering figures of twentieth-century health policy and management. Bob Sigmond reviewed the book for the publisher and subsequently met with us on two memorable occasions. Those who know Bob will appreciate how stimulating these meetings were. We are in debt to him not only for his time and wisdom but for his belief in the importance of health capital and community planning and for his willingness to wade into the complex details of institutional design.

Capital research and policy constitute only one of the many areas in which Dr. Rorem broke new ground and literally "wrote the book" during his career. It was an honor as well as a great pleasure to meet him in New Jersey to receive his comments on the manuscript firsthand.

I wonder why familial acknowledgments are always saved until last. In the larger scheme of things they come and always will come first. My wife, Jan-Lee Betz, and our children, Henry Charles Betz Brown and Sarah Jeanne Betz Brown, know–doubtless better than I–the great thanks they deserve. I trust they also know how much I value them. I put this book to bed with the words I often hear when Sarah wakes me up: "I love you so-o-o-o much!"

NOTES

1. Health policy analysts often call health providers "hammers looking for a nail." So are we all. I await the day when university faculty are subjected to the same withering forces of analysis and rationalization that they have directed with such smugness at the doctors.
2. Benjamin R. Barber, *Strong Democracy: Participatory Politics for a New Age* (Berkeley: University of California Press, 1984), p. 254. Emphasis in the original.

INTRODUCTION

Over the next decade, the United States will invest hundreds of billions of dollars of capital in health-related buildings, equipment, programs, and firms. This money will finance a wide range of institutions: multinational for-profit health care corporations and struggling neighborhood health centers led by community boards, public hospitals that serve our poorest citizens and free-standing ambulatory surgery centers in wealthy suburbs, 50-bed rural hospitals and 500-bed academic medical centers, programs to prevent infant mortality and ultrasophisticated neonatal intensive care units, "life-care" communities that combine real estate development with long-term care insurance and hospices for the terminally ill, programs to combat drug abuse and for-profit clinics that sell patients the chance to test new drugs. Where this capital flows will determine the physical shape and strongly influence the equity and effectiveness of the future health care system. If we invest intelligently, future capital investment choices can make the health care system much more productive, more accessible, and more humane. Tens of thousands of excess acute hospital beds, profiteering in the nursing home industry, and decaying hospitals in poor neighborhoods show what can happen if we do not. Either way, future capital investment will affect how long we live and the quality of our days.

As citizens, employers, and users of services, we not only depend on this investment, we will pay for it. We will pay through health insurance premiums: our premiums provide much of the revenue that hospitals and other institutions spend to build facilities and buy equipment, pledge to repay construction loans, and distribute to shareholders. We will lend the money and buy the stocks that finance major construction. We will pay the taxes that support Medicare and Medicaid and that subsidize tax exemptions for voluntary hospitals, many health maintenance organizations, Blue Cross and Blue Shield plans, and purchasers of tax-exempt bonds. Rarely, it appears, will anyone ask how we would like our money invested.

In this book, we ask. More important, we ask how to ask, by studying whether a democratic institution capable of planning a portion of U.S. health capital investment could be designed. We ask because we are worried. Capital payment policies proposed for the coming competitive era are more apt to destabilize the system than to guide it. The federal Medicare program is preparing to end cost-based capital reimbursement of hospitals by folding capital reimbursement into the preset prices it pays for hospital admissions. Health maintenance organizations (HMOs) and other care managers do the same thing when they negotiate private contracts with hospitals, physicians, and clinics. Such arrangements make an institution's ability to raise capital almost entirely dependent on its ability to make a profit.

This imperative to profit will influence care-giving behavior since, in the long run, institutional survival depends on access to capital. Moreover, the revenues institutions receive will more and more be dictated by large purchasers of care – monopsonists is the proper economic term – and relentless downward pressure on revenues is likely to result. Already, a large fraction – perhaps a majority – of hospitals in the United States could not get access to bond markets should they wish to rebuild, and many institutions in poor neighborhoods have failed. Large, for-profit companies, which for several reasons enjoy much greater access to capital than freestanding voluntary institutions, may join with nominally nonprofit institutions that have abandoned their social mission in an effort to dominate health care wherever it is profitable. Health care may again become segregated by class and race. Opportunities for consumer and business influence and control over health care may vanish. For many of us, the health care vessel we have come to rely upon may capsize.

For four years, participants in Harvard University's Health Capital Project wrestled with these problems and explored the possibilities for health capital payment reform. We have come to appreciate how central a role capital has played in past attempts to support and coordinate health system behavior. For regulators, capital investment has provided a target that is visible, accessible, and important. For community leaders, capital funds are an essential resource which, at times, they have controlled. For hospitals and other institutions, both physical capital and financial capital are resources they cannot live without.

We also came to realize that, in a competitive health economic environment, capital payment reform and other capital policies should not be evaluated or designed in isolation. Broader policies and trends—the encouragement of competition or expanded entitlement for the uninsured, for example—affect capital access and investment at least as strongly as explicit capital policies like certificate of need (CoN) or tax exemption for hospital bonds. Similarly, capital funds and physical capital expenditures are not the only health resources that unaided competitive markets will fail to manage effectively. Capital is a prominent member of a class of resources and services that require explicit public management, at least in part, if true equity and efficiency are to be approximated. In some cases, such as medical care for the homeless, no market exists without governmental intervention. In other cases, such as hospital renovation and construction, private markets may work in well-to-do areas but fail in poor and rural areas. As we recognized this truth and broadened our horizons accordingly, we came to see our job as the design of a public management structure for an entire *cooperative sector* that encompasses all the resources and services that private markets cannot manage on their own.

We have a modest proposal. Or, more accurately, we outline the basic framework of an institution—we call it a community health infrastructure bank, or CHIB—which state governments and communities can adapt to make policy and manage resources in the cooperative sector. A CHIB offers a way for communities to purchase services and invest in buildings, equipment, and programs that market mechanisms fail to supply. Stripped to its essentials, a CHIB pools funds and reallocates them to achieve community objectives.

Health care leaders beginning with Michael Davis, the founder in 1934 of the first U.S. graduate program in hospital administration, and C. Rufus Rorem, the developer of the original Blue Cross plans in the 1930s, have advocated capital pooling. However, hospitals opposed pooling once guaranteed reimbursement for capital and operating expenditures made most hospitals self-sufficient borrowers of funds. We revitalize and extend this old debate in two directions. First, we show how the idea of capital pooling can be adapted to the competitive economic structures and philosophies of the future. In the process, we show how pooling differs fundamentally from historical forms of capital investment regulation, including certificate of need, and from the prevalent kind of health planning that discourages innovation and entrepreneurial initiative. Second, we examine in detail just how pooling might be made to work. The CHIB model we present emerges from a serious consideration of the reasons for the lack of political accountability, constructive incentives, competent management, and strategic vision that hindered health planning in the past. Pooling itself offers the best framework for solving many of these problems.

In writing this book we came to see our task as the design of an institution capable of planning and managing resources for an entire cooperative sector. We focus on health capital policy because of its intrinsic importance and because it was our starting point. However, capital also offers an excellent tracer or case example that highlights design issues of relevance throughout the cooperative sector. Thus, before introducing our CHIB design in detail, we devote Chapter 1 to a description and analysis of the U.S. health capital policies of the recent and more distant past. This history, while not widely known or appreciated in health policy and management circles, is instructive. It shows how health capital exerts its great strategic influence over the character and development of the health care system and how a surprisingly wide range of policies affect the acquisition and use of capital in health. It also teaches the futility of attempting to design or evaluate capital policies without carefully considering the larger policy and economic environments in which they operate. It reminds us that hospitals and other health service delivery institutions only recently became independent of philanthropy as a source of capital and community control. This era of commercial independence may turn out to have been only a temporary departure from a longer run pattern of public control.[1]

In Chapter 2, we briefly forecast the health system environment of the future and explain why well-planned capital policies will be needed to offset its adverse aspects. We then evaluate the widely admired capital payment alternative, flat-rate or market capital payment. We find little to admire, as the brief discussion earlier in this introduction indicates, although Medicare and other payers may adopt this form of payment in the years to come. Our predictions about future health system evolution and the effects of market payment, however, help us understand what alternative payment systems must be designed to do.

Then, in Chapter 3, we begin a consideration of how an alternative or complementary system, planned payment, might be organized. We review the history of prior attempts to implement planned payment, including the popular Hill-Burton program and the efforts of successful early "business coalitions" during the 1960s. We extract from these examples important lessons that help us identify prerequisites for successful planned payment. We compare such a program to certificate of need, a much different policy in both structure and intent, but the one most persons think of when they hear the term, planned payment. We show how most of the defects that cause CoN's ineffectiveness and unpopularity are remedied in a properly designed planned payment system operating in a more competitive health care environment.

By Chapter 4 we are ready to begin designing a specific planned payment arrangement, the community health infrastructure bank. In this chapter, we identify and discuss key design decisions, including sources of funding, forms of allocation, management and planning systems, and organization structure. We continue the analysis in Chapter 5, with a discussion of how a CHIB should be governed and how it should relate to existing governmental and voluntary organizations. We opt, in Chapter 5, for a governmental organization led by an independent board, but one more accountable than most independent boards to gubernatorial authority.

In Chapter 6, we reflect on the organization we have proposed and consider the historical forces and tactics that could move it off the drawing board and into use. Surprisingly, the flat-rate capital payment mechanisms being adopted by Medicare and other payers—although the philosophical antithesis of planned payment in the minds of many of its supporters—should make CHIBs more attractive and easier to finance. The spread of competition in health services markets and the fiscal crisis of the federal government also should spur interest and support. If, in the longer run, the nation turns away from competition and toward more centralized health financing structures like those of Canada and Europe, CHIBs can provide an effective foundation on which to build.

The entire U.S. health care system appears to be changing now toward a new, competitive structure composed of insurers who actively manage our care and providers who compete to sell them services. The change may vastly improve both equity and efficiency, or it may squander in a few years a public investment in buildings, equipment, people, and institutions that the nation took a century to create. We believe that, as a sailboat's keel provides stability and allows the boat to be steered, the health capital policy of the future should be designed to stabilize and guide health care through the heavy seas ahead—help it catch the winds of change, maintain headway, and avoid the shoals.

In the final analysis, this book is about much more than health capital policy and a particular problem in institutional design. It represents an attempt to see clearly the semicompetitive health care environment now being created in the United States and to develop public responses that go beyond either ideological cheer leading or reactionary, sentimental debunking. We try to identify a public policy that shores up the good qualities of the emerging competition and protects the integrity that markets need to be effective, while ameliorating competition's adverse side effects and developing an effective nonmarket institution to manage the problems it cannot handle.

Academics and policy makers spend a good deal of time – although probably not enough – considering how markets can be structured to make competition work in health. But markets, no matter how well designed, will never provide a total solution. We need to spend as much time, or more time, in designing complementary *political* institutions that can also be successful. This book makes an early contribution to this effort.

NOTE

1. The preoccupation in U.S. health policy with markets and competition tends to make terms like *public*, *governmental*, and *community* seem synonymous. They are not. In this book, when we talk about public management of resources, we refer to auspices that may be entirely governmental, entirely voluntary (nongovernmental), or anything in between. Public simply means that individuals act together consciously through political institutions, broadly defined, rather than through markets. The term *community* reinforces the idea of geographic location implicit in the word *public* and reminds us that health for all residents of an area is the goal that most Americans expect their health system to pursue. We use *community* broadly in this book to refer to areas as small as towns or as large as states. We assume that communities can act through a variety of public institutions.

1.

Health Capital Policy: The Long View

Capital exerts great influence in health care, as in the rest of the economy. This is true although private investors own only a minority of health service delivery capacity in the United States. The influence of capital persists for several reasons.

First, not-for-profit as well as proprietary (for-profit) hospitals, nursing homes, health centers, home care providers, and other service delivery organizations need safe and efficient buildings and up-to-date equipment. They also need working capital to finance operations until clients and insurance companies pay their bills and to meet other operational needs. Organizations need additional capital to start new services and finance organizational change, and to cope with developments in their operating environment such as changes in technology, disease patterns, consumer preferences, regulatory and reimbursement programs, and competition from other providers.

No health delivery institution can survive in the long run without access to capital funds to meet these various needs. Health care institutions, therefore, tend to tailor themselves to the expectations of the individuals and institutions that can provide capital. They adapt or fail. During the twentieth century, U.S. hospitals have transformed their mission and management more than once to accommodate changing sources of capital and operating revenue.

Capital-adaptive behavior helps determine, in turn, what health services society receives and the cost, quality, and accessibility of these services. For example, past capital commitments tend to lock up future earnings and lock in configurations of service production capacity.

Future earnings are locked up in part because health institutions nearly always finance major new construction and renovation with long-term borrowing, which must be repaid with interest. In addition, for acute care hospitals, the life-cycle operating costs associated with new buildings and equipment typically exceed purchase costs by a factor of 20 or so.[1] Of course, no law requires that capital be utilized once it is purchased, but it tends to be. As a result, capital investment determines the consumption of much of the discretionary resource available to the health system and channels health system evolution and planning. It affects both the capacity to produce services and the character of the services produced.

Once delivery institutions convert financial capital into "bricks and mortar," equipment, and new services, these physical assets and programmatic commitments assume a life of their own. Hospitals, especially, find it difficult to shift buildings and equipment to other uses. When they can, the cost of conversion is often great, and profits from successor uses may not repay debt service plus conversion costs. (Commercial and manufacturing space, by contrast, enjoys active rental and resale markets.) Physical capital commitments thus "set in concrete" much of the future physical configuration of the health care system.

The changing interactions among sources of health capital, sources of operating revenue, and hospital behavior since 1900 demonstrate, as no abstract analysis can, the fundamental strategic importance of health capital policy. An understanding of this history—a history not widely known in current health policy circles—provides such a useful starting point for an analysis of future health capital policy that we begin our book by describing it. Surprisingly, unintentional and indirect policies play a more prominent role in this history than many policies aimed directly at health capital behavior; hence, our description focuses primarily on the interaction between hospital behavior and health services financing and reimbursement. We postpone a discussion of certificate of need (CoN) and related governmental efforts to plan and regulate capital expenditures—efforts that were largely ineffective—until the conclusion of the chapter. We do describe at its proper chronological point the brief "golden age" of voluntary health planning that occurred in some cities during the early 1960s, but we omit any detailed account of the Hill-Burton program—another partial success—until Chapter 3. Chapter 3 also contains a more detailed analysis of certificate of need and federally mandated health planning.

1900–1931: THE ERA OF PERSONAL PHILANTHROPY

The first great expansion of hospital capacity during the twentieth century occurred in the United States between 1900 and about 1930. The ranks of hospitals of all kinds swelled from slightly over 2,000 in 1900 to nearly 7,000 in 1928.[2] More than 4,500 of these were general hospitals, including 1,889 not-for-profit (voluntary) hospitals, 1,877 for-profit (proprietary) and industrial hospitals, and 772 government facilities.[3] Because they were larger than proprietary institutions, voluntary hospitals accounted for a majority of the general hospital beds.

A key element of health capital policy during this period was the belief that government should restrict its managerial involvement largely to institutions designed to isolate dangerous or unpleasant citizens from the community. Government thus operated tuberculosis sanatoria, mental hospitals, and a few general hospitals that served society's most marginal members. Acute general hospitals by and large sought capitalization from private sources, which for voluntary hospitals during this period meant wealthy individual donors. Towns also contributed through local government grants. Voluntary hospitals subsidized the costs of treating indigent and "part-pay" patients by raising charges to middle- and upper-class patients. Local community chests, wealthy trustees, and local government paid any remaining shortfalls.

A large number of proprietary hospitals emerged and appear to have flourished during this period. Unlike the proprietary institutions of today, they were financed by individual physician owners, often with philanthropic help. Most were located in towns and rural areas (where the vast majority of Americans lived during this period) and functioned much like voluntary community hospitals. Physician owners hoped to make up in their practice the funds they often lost in operating the hospital. In fact, it was common for such facilities to move back and forth between proprietary and voluntary ownership depending on financial circumstances and physician movement. In urban areas with many general hospitals, some proprietaries limited their services to paying patients and may have attracted business by keeping their prices below the artificially high rates established by cross-subsidizing voluntaries.

Although communities often subsidized hospital operations either by making up annual shortfalls or by appropriating governmental funds to support indigent patients on a per diem basis, operating cost recovery was based primarily on a commercial relationship between patients and institutions. (In Europe, by contrast, hospitals developed as givers rather than sellers of services.[4]) Paradoxically, however, *capital* finance for most general hospital beds in the United States depended not on market economics but on the *charity* of wealthy donors.

The fact that market relationships generated operating revenues while donors financed capital decreased operating efficiency and diminished the effectiveness of capital donations during this period. In his path-breaking 1930 study, *The Public's Investment in Hospitals,* C. Rufus Rorem observed that

> [m]any hospital superintendents [administrators] have taken no part in the financing or the construction of the plant and equipment which are under their control. Their administrative efficiency has generally been judged by their ability to balance cash budgets for operating costs. . . . [O]nce a hospital has been built, a superintendent may improve the cash position of his budget by caring for convalescent or long-term patients in the existing accommodation rather than by providing new ones specially adapted for these services. One may expect to find, therefore, that although there is much discussion at the present time of the need for convalescent and rest facilities, some hospitals with unfilled beds will not wish to lose the class of patients for which operating costs are the lowest.[5]

The separation of capital planning and operating management thus not only created adverse incentives for operating managers but made it more difficult to target new capital investment effectively.

Rorem also noticed that uncoordinated funding by private donors was inefficient and unreliable: "Rather than wound the vanity of a wealthy donor, certain [larger] communities have accepted facilities which were essentially monuments to his pride instead of stations of public welfare."[6] In addition, in urban areas, rival independent associations or churches would often vie with each other in administering to the public needs, resulting in duplication and the establishment of hospitals too small to operate efficiently.

Rorem advocated restrictions on donations for hospital construction in order to free up funds for other social needs, including the subsidization of free hospital care, which typically ran a poor second to erecting new edifices in the minds of individual donors.[7] Observing that most new investment in hospitals by 1928 was for renovation and improvement rather than expansion or new facilities ("intensification" was his word), Rorem thought future capital needs could be better met by regular annual contributions to institutional depreciation accounts. (Hospitals at this time did not maintain depreciation accounts, and few kept records of their physical assets.) Rorem hoped the growing community chest movement, which helped finance the operating deficits but not the major capital needs of most voluntary hospitals, might finance and allocate these contributions.

> If community chests, and doctors and hospitals participating in their planning, were to change their policies and definitely set out to control hospital construction, and also to raise funds for plant and equipment, much good might be accomplished. The prevention of duplication of hospital facilities might release much capital for the current subsidizing of hospital care.[8]

But, Rorem was realistic enough to add, "[t]his method is not in contemplation by most community chests and may not become an integral part of their policies within the near future,"[9] as indeed it did not.[10] Hospitals did eventually adopt his accounting reforms after World War II, however, once hospital insurance became widespread and third-party payers began to reimburse capital expenses on the basis of cost.

1932–1945: PUBLIC FINANCING TAKES OVER

The Great Depression and subsequent wartime shortages of materials abruptly reduced the problem of unnecessary investment in voluntary and proprietary hospitals. Nevertheless, during the years of economic hardship, local government combined with philanthropy to increase the flow of capital gifts and operating subsidies. Communities apparently assumed responsibility for the operation of many financially pressed rural and small-town proprietary hospitals at this time. Although voluntary agencies increased the absolute value of their contributions to all hospitals throughout the depression, from 1928 to 1935 an increasing proportion of investment in hospitals came from government.[11] The federal government, acting through the Public Works Administration, the Work Projects Administration, the Reconstruction Finance Corporation, and other agencies, funded considerable construction during the 1930s and early 1940s:[12] more than 2,500 hospital projects and hundreds of hospitals. Governmental funds were allocated primarily to hospitals owned and operated by county or local government, rather than to voluntary or proprietary institutions, however. By 1939, public hospital construction subsidies exceeded private funds by a ratio of four to one.

Local government hospitals served a pressing need. In large cities these were the institutions to which the unemployed turned when hard-pressed voluntary hospitals, whose solvency depended on paying patients, could not afford to treat them. The 1938 Hospital Survey of New York contrasted an overcrowded municipal hospital system with a voluntary system saddled with large numbers of empty beds.[13] The trustees of the city's voluntary hospitals created the nation's first prominent voluntary health planning agency, the Hospital Council of Greater New York, to try to reverse this imbalance.[14]

The decision of federal policy makers to route economic recovery aid through governmental organizations, coupled with the lack of any universal system to pay for the care of indigent patients in voluntary and private hospitals, reinforced a two-class system of hospital and medical care in urban areas. Again during the 1930s, health capital policy, acting in conjunction with policies affecting operating cost recovery, contributed to fundamental change in health system structure and trajectory.

1946–1966: NEW SOURCES OF CAPITAL AND A BRIEF SUCCESS FOR PLANNING

The Rise of Insurance and Governmental Grants-in-Aid

More voluntary hospitals might have closed during the depression had not C. Rufus Rorem and others promoted the establishment of systems for voluntary prepayment of hospital services. Initially, these plans developed as combined capitation-service benefit contracts between individual hospitals and enrollees: for a given monthly contribution, say 50 cents, a hospital would agree to provide up to a specified amount of comprehensive nonphysician hospital services, say 21 days of semiprivate care. By 1932, however,

> a multiplicity of individual hospital-sponsored payment plans began to interfere with freedom of choice of physician and hospital, since any subscriber would naturally insist on going to the hospital to which he was making monthly payments. . . . In addition, the inefficiency of separate enrollment drives became evident. As a consequence of these two factors, multihospital plans—soon to be called Blue Cross—came into being. . . . There was only one small change that did not seem too important at the time: The basis of payment *to the hospital* was changed from *per subscriber* (sick and well alike) to *per diem* for those subscribers who were patients.[15]

By 1945, an estimated 30 million Americans (22 percent of the population) were enrolled in some type of voluntary prepayment or health insurance plan.[16] Although the Kaiser Foundation Health Plan and some other health maintenance organizations (HMOs) founded during this era continued to use per-subscriber payment, the shift to per diem payment was to have profoundly negative effects on health care finance and delivery for many years to come. It was not until the 1980s that alternative approaches began to see widespread use.

In addition, the federal Emergency Maternity and Infant Care program (EMIC) began in March 1943 to finance pregnancy and perinatal care for families of enlisted men. EMIC appears to have been the first major hospital financing program to require hospitals to submit statements of actual operating costs and to use these statements to calculate reimbursement. (Blue Cross plans did not use cost-based reimbursement "because of the unwillingness of hospitals to make available actual costs of furnishing hospital service,"[17] and because of wide variation in accounting methods. Instead, most Blue Cross plans until 1969 negotiated flat per diem rates.[18]) EMIC also was the first financing program to reimburse explicitly for capital costs: a generous 10 percent was added to per diem payments to cover depreciation, rent, and interest.[19]

When the Commission on Hospital Care published its encyclopedic survey of hospitals and hospital affairs in 1947,[20] philanthropy still provided most capital funds and subsidized operating losses in most voluntary hospitals, and hospital accounting remained rudimentary. But a movement toward financing capital needs from operating revenues had begun. Also about this time, in 1945, Congress amended the tax code to allow businesses to deduct, from income, contributions to agencies that sought to improve the general standards of a community. By 1947, corporate gifts accounted for roughly 15 percent of gifts to hospital capital drives, a percentage that was to increase dramatically in the years to come.[21]

The post–World War II period also witnessed the creation and subsequent expansion of the Hospital Survey and Construction Act of 1946, known popularly as the Hill-Burton program. A complex and influential program, Hill-Burton was drafted by leaders of the U.S. Public Health Service (PHS) and "approved line by line by the American Hospital Association" (AHA).[22] It distributed more than $3 billion in federal funds to nonprofit hospitals and long-term care facilities by 1968 and stimulated a matching investment of $7 billion in primarily private funds: philanthropy, debt, internal reserves, and, occasionally, state governmental funding. Proprietary hospitals were excluded from participation. Spending associated with Hill-Burton accounted for 40 percent of the $24.6 billion expended on health facilities construction during this period, much of it construction that might not otherwise have been undertaken.[23]

In its early years, Hill-Burton provided construction grants and loans to voluntary and public hospitals in rural areas that lacked modern acute care beds. Although Congress gave considerable discretion to the line governmental agencies that implemented the program in each state, it created national standards of need that were simplistic, formulaic, and intentionally overly generous. Many small rural hospitals were built that would later prove inefficient, insolvent, and—many believed—unsafe. As Congress continued to fund the program at increasing levels, suburban and then certain urban hospitals became major beneficiaries, along with a range of nonhospital facilities; for many financially secure hospitals, access to program funds became a question more of "when" than of "whether." We describe the Hill-Burton program in detail and analyze its strengths and weaknesses in Chapter 3.

Despite this massive investment of public funds, the period from the middle 1940s to the middle 1960s witnessed an increasing substitution of commercial values and behavior for community service and community control of hospital and medical care. The growing percentage of Americans participating in hospital insurance and prepayment plans, which rose from 33 percent in 1945 to 57 percent in 1965,[24] meant that, increasingly, hospitals could achieve at least partial financial independence from Hill-Burton and philanthropy.

Moreover, these payers were willing to recognize capital expenditure as a routine cost of doing business: Blue Cross plans typically included a flat-rate capital allowance in the contracts they negotiated with hospitals, and hospitals included amounts for depreciation and interest when they calculated the charges that commercial insurers and private-pay patients paid. By increasing operating revenues to cover capital requirements, hospitals began to imitate for-profit enterprises which, broadly speaking, maintain capital depreciation accounts in order to preserve and increase the capital investment of their owners.

For-profit enterprises, however, move capital from business to business and from location to location in pursuit of profit, and stockholders shift their own funds from firm to firm. By demanding payment for depreciation and interest, immobile community hospitals implicitly assumed that communities would benefit by their perpetual recapitalization regardless of future changes in technology, population, disease, or their own performance. Such an attitude might be justified if hospitals saw themselves as guardians of community health and behaved accordingly; if they took responsibility for the health of the population rather than simply providing a workshop for fee-for-service physicians; if they actively studied community epidemiology and based their planning on priority community needs; if they aggressively sought to care for the uninsured, to coordinate services with other institutions rather than duplicate them, to educate their communities, to monitor aggressively and manage their own quality and utilization, and to provide preventive, environmental, and occupational health services.

A few hospitals made notable attempts to take community health seriously. Most others provided some free care to indigent patients. But, by and large, hospitals were not in a position to assume responsibility for the health of the population.[25] They were created to provide a fairly narrow range of curative services, and their economic survival depended on their ability to provide an attractive workshop for their fee-for-service physicians, most of whom adamantly opposed any "socialistic" conception of public duty. In an increasingly overbedded environment, they actively competed among themselves to attract physicians who would bring more patients and greater revenues. Often the competition took the form of capital investment: new facilities in wealthy suburban neighborhoods, the latest technology and equipment, and nearby medical office buildings.

Hospital revenues continued to increase during the 1950s and early 1960s. The per diem paid by Blue Cross plans grew rapidly, prompting public outcry and leading eventually to a rationalization of Blue Cross payment principles on the basis of historical-cost reimbursement, fund accounting, and modern overhead apportionment methods. But the now widely recognized cost-generating incentives of per diem, historical-cost reimbursement added fuel to the cost inflation fire, as did the growing share of the insured population enrolled in charge-paying commercial insurance plans. Commercial insurers dealt with rising costs not by questioning their payments to hospitals but by limiting their total liability per enrollee. They kept their premium prices low by "experience rating"–seeking out enrollee groups that were less likely on average to incur large hospital bills. Ultimately, commercial competition encouraged nearly all the nation's Blue Cross plans to abandon the alternative approach, "community rating," by which group enrollees in an area paid equal premiums regardless of their probable cost to the plan. As nonprofit corporations, chartered by special state legislative acts and governed by community leaders, Blue Cross began with a conception of medical care as a social good and with a commitment to redistribute premiums on the basis of social need. Experience rating put Blue Cross organizations on a much more commercial footing.

Competition from commercial insurers probably also discouraged the Blues from using their influence to regulate hospital revenues and encourage community service.[26] Not only were the Blue Cross plans' market shares small in many areas, but the opportunity for hospitals to extract extra revenues from the charge-paying commercials allowed Blue Cross plans to keep their own per diem payments, which were established by contracts that included special discounts, lower than the competition. Absent a general social revolt, most Blue Cross plans had little commercial incentive to limit the growing insulation of hospitals from community concerns and control.

Despite their growing potential for financial independence, most hospitals did not actually fund depreciation accounts or manage their costs with an eye toward accumulating savings. Although third-party payers accounted for fully 80 percent of hospital revenue by 1960,[27] even as late as 1965 hospitals still financed about 50 percent of major construction projects from philanthropy,[28] which by this time came largely from local corporations. Borrowing was on the rise but still constituted less than 16 percent of non-church-related voluntary hospital construction financing:[29] banks and other lenders knew that revenues were uncertain and that both economic barriers (no resale market) and political reaction would make it difficult to foreclose hospital mortgages.[30] Nevertheless, the increasingly comfortable reimbursement environment whetted hospitals' appetites for investment, as did the technical advance of curative medicine, rising wages and gross national product, rapid population growth in and around cities, and changes in the Hill-Burton program.[31] As a decade-long boom in hospital construction gathered momentum, corporate leaders in some communities realized that the combined capital ambitions of their individual hospitals would far outstrip both community need and corporate willingness to pay. In response, a "golden age" of voluntary areawide planning flowered briefly, based on the ability of organized donors to control the funds that hospitals were able to invest.

Planning's Golden Age

In towns like Rochester, Pittsburgh, and Detroit, where a concentrated and often paternalistic corporate structure facilitated cooperation, business and community leaders began to review hospital capital investment plans and encourage hospitals to take a community-oriented approach to the development and management of services. Foundations like the Commonwealth Fund and the W.K. Kellogg Foundation began to lay the groundwork for this effort as early as the 1940s by financing areawide planning efforts and hospital construction.[32] The U.S. Public Health Service provided financial and intellectual support to such areawide planning efforts, starting in 1959. After Hill-Burton began to subsidize planning agencies in 1962, new "hospital planning councils," as they were usually called, appeared at the rate of about 10 per year.[33] The economist Herbert Klarman counted 63 hospital planning councils in 1966, 55 of which had been organized in the previous four years.[34]

A particularly successful council in Rochester, New York took charge of a citywide hospital capital fund drive in 1960 and trimmed hospital requests from $30 million to $14 million. As a result of this assertion of community control, Rochester held its bed-to-population ratio to 3.4 per 1,000, a rate that proved the envy of less provident cities for decades to come. In addition, taking advantage of the freedom of action provided by their pool of capital funds, the community representatives closed a low-quality proprietary hospital as well as an inadequate county chronic disease hospital and established new institutions that guaranteed much better care for the displaced patients.[35] Community control also resulted in the establishment in Rochester of intermediate care facilities and other innovations, the need for which was identified by communitywide epidemiologic studies.[36]

In Pittsburgh, the Hospital Planning Association of Allegheny County got started when the Hospital Council of Western Pennsylvania surveyed its membership in the late 1950s. As in Rochester, the council discovered that each institution had capital investment plans that, in the aggregate, greatly exceeded any reasonable definition of community need or ability to pay. Eighteen of the area's largest corporations donated funds toward a study of how to coordinate these capital proposals, and that study led to the association's establishment.

> [I]t was recognized that effective planning involves the ability to say "no," a capability that hopefully need never be exercised. Nevertheless, if the Hospital Council was to do the planning, there was the risk that important hospitals would pull out in response to negative reactions to their plans. This would tear the Council apart. Alternatively, if ability to say "no" was not exercised, everyone would be scratching everyone else's back and the whole thing would be a waste of time.
>
> The decision was reached to set up an independent organization; and so that it should have the power to say "no," it ought to represent the power in the community. In Pittsburgh that's not the government. It's the corporations. . . . I think some of our hospitals would rather have seen some government participation so that it might be a little more wishy-washy. But the corporations put up most of the money for hospital buildings and they were asked to get the organization going. Its board of directors includes the heads of all the largest corporations in the Pittsburgh area.[37]

The first executive director of the association was C. Rufus Rorem. He and his successors—Robert M. Sigmond, first, then Steven Sieverts—took the view that creating the preconditions for action was more important than writing master plans. As a major element in this strategy, they sought to create, *within each hospital,* the capacity to plan for *community* needs. They viewed the hospital as the natural base from which to develop community health services. Each hospital was asked to develop a service plan based on careful epidemiologic analysis. The association provided data, technical assistance, and constant encouragement. But, as hospitals gained the financial independence to ignore the association when it said no,[38] the association seems to have relied more and more on efforts to facilitate internal institutional planning. By 1968, Sieverts wrote,

> [w]here the system has broken down, it is largely because of inadequate . . . planning at the institutional level. If we can blame the existence of two side-by-side under-used and ineffectively staffed cobalt-therapy installa-

tions on poor planning by the two hospitals, isn't improving their planning a better solution than just forbidding one of the installations?[39]

Rochester's community leaders appear to have had greater impact because they controlled an actual pool of funds–the major source of hospital capital funding during the period of their success. Large corporations were not the only economic actors that controlled capital funds or that shared an economic incentive to limit their use. Local Blue Cross plans also made significant payments–indeed, the era of financial stability that Blue Cross ushered in allowed hospitals to begin their escape from philanthropic control–and Blue Cross suffered competitively and politically from cost inflation induced by excess capacity. In a landmark 1962 survey and analysis entitled *Hospital and Medical Economics,* Walter J. McNerny and William R. Foyle recommended that

> Blue Cross contribute to the capital needs of hospitals by placing in trust, or trusts established geographically, an amount based on the number of subscribers without relation to the area's hospitals, their volume, or cost of services; and that management of the trust or trusts be vested in a trustee and expenditure of these funds be the responsibility of a state hospital commission.[40]

McNerny and Foyle also suggested that "hospitals would probably benefit by pooling depreciation funds in a common trust fund . . . managed by a bank or trust company."[41]

Robert Sigmond went further. In a 1964 speech to the American Hospital Association, Sigmond observed that

> [a]ny obligation to preserve the public's investment in hospitals as the plants wear out does not imply an obligation to preserve the public's investment in each hospital *at each hospital*. . . . Blue Cross and other contracting agencies can pay most effectively for the capital their beneficiaries consume by contributing a sum to the hospital system, based on their share of the depreciation of the hospital system. Placed in a pooled fund, this money could be a significant source of capital. It could be spent annually or whenever needed by those hospitals that have well developed, community-oriented modernization programs. . . . In a period in which so much capital is needed, it is tragic to "sterilize" large amounts of money in individual hospital depreciation accounts.[42]

Sigmond also called on hospitals to turn back from increasing reliance on debt and other commercial sources of funds. However, few hospital administrators supported Sigmond's proposal, fearing loss of control of "their" funds. Sigmond "lost many friends"[43] in the hospital industry, and areawide planning in Pittsburgh "suffered a major setback."[44]

Subsequent efforts to establish planned payment mechanisms also met defeat. By the late 1960s, at least one Blue Cross plan in New Jersey reduced the reimbursement rate of any hospital that added beds without receiving planning council approval, by "the amount such expansion adds to the rate."[45] In some other states, unapproved expansion could result in loss of the hospital's Blue Cross contract.[46] Walter J. McNerny, who became president of the national Blue Cross Association, threatened in 1968 to force similar actions nationwide. But, as McNerny was later to remark, "Fresh out of Ann Arbor, I had a lot of ideas about how to improve the delivery system through the financing process. A fair number of those ideas ended up as polite policy statements, or worse, as exhortations."[47]

The planned payment idea suffered a similar fate when Congress considered legislation that would require hospitals to fund their depreciation accounts and prohibit expenditures from the funds for big-ticket capital projects that were not approved by local planning agencies. Despite bipartisan support and provisions that would have allowed borrowing from the account (the majority of hospitals used depreciation payments to meet operating expenses), the initiative was not enacted.

Instead, easy access to capital and the prospect of economic independence attracted hospital administrators to the possibility of including capital costs in contract rates and prices. The American Hospital Association had long supported areawide planning in publications and policy statements. In 1969, the AHA endorsed a weak variant of planned capital payment in its new *Statement on the Financial Requirements of Health Care Institutions and Services*. In addition to asking for historical-cost reimbursement for depreciation, and for new and additional payments to amortize the principal and interest of existing debt, the AHA asked Blue Cross and other contract payers to pay their pro rata share of the costs of all new capital investment recommended for approval by a local planning agency. The identity of the planning agency was to be specified in private contracts with the payers.

Despite its apparent support for community planning of investment, this *Statement* marked the end of hospital reliance on community-controlled sources of capital. Medicare and Blue Cross plans, the latter facing increasing competitive pressure from commercial insurers, balked at paying more than depreciation and interest on debt, an approach the AHA had recommended in earlier statements on financial requirements. But these payments were enough, when combined with the surpluses hospitals earned from their charge-paying patients, to give hospitals financial independence—or, more precisely, to substitute market discipline for the possibility of a measure of community control. Hospitals are only now beginning to look back.

1967–1987: HOSPITALS GO IT ALONE

Almost as soon as they had seized control of capital–and therefore of hospital behavior–communities found their control beginning to slip away. After weakening the basic allocation formula in 1962 to loosen bed supply controls and favor growing suburban areas, Congress in 1964 doubled Hill-Burton appropriations and made funds available for renovation and modernization as well as new construction. Simultaneously, the ability of hospitals to borrow on the strength of their own future operating revenues increased dramatically. Whereas nonsectarian voluntary hospitals borrowed 16 percent of construction financing in 1965, they borrowed 40 percent in 1969; by 1973, about 60 percent came from debt.[48] And although philanthropy continued to grow in absolute terms, as a percentage of construction financing it became dwarfed by debt, Hill-Burton, and the dramatic growth in total health facility construction activity–a 250 percent jump from $1.5 billion to $3.8 billion per year between 1960 and 1970.[49] As Robert M. Sigmond put it, "Increasingly, the traditional fund drive . . . is carried out primarily, if at all, for its public relations value rather than for money-raising purposes."[50]

The event that suddenly allowed hospitals to borrow much more heavily was the enactment of the Medicare and Medicaid programs in 1965, along with the negotiations over Medicare payment practices that preceded that program's implementation in July 1966. The story is a complex and fascinating one, well told by several authors.[51] The key outcomes from the standpoint of health system development and capital policy were two. First, Medicare and Medicaid converted most of the average hospital's nonpaying patients into paying patients. This greatly increased hospital financial stability.

Second, decisions were made about the regulations governing Medicare hospital payment that colored access to capital and health system development for nearly two decades. It was decided to pay for operating costs retrospectively on the basis of actual costs incurred, to meet capital needs by recognizing and reimbursing interest expense and depreciation at actual historical cost, and–at the last minute–to give proprietary institutions a generous allowance for return on investor equity.[52] The American Hospital Association then wrote these arrangements into its *Statement on the Financial Requirements of Health Care Institutions and Services* as minimum standards of payment and secured capital reimbursement on similar (or better) terms from some Blue Cross plans. In effect, the nation's hospitals gave themselves the financial security to enter private debt and equity markets and to control their own destinies much like commercial enterprises. The autonomy-creating effect of this security far outweighed the two major restrictive effects of the shift to

Exhibit 1-1
Medical Facilities Construction and Third-Party Payments to Hospitals, as a Percentage of Total U.S. Hospital Expenditures, 1950 to 1984

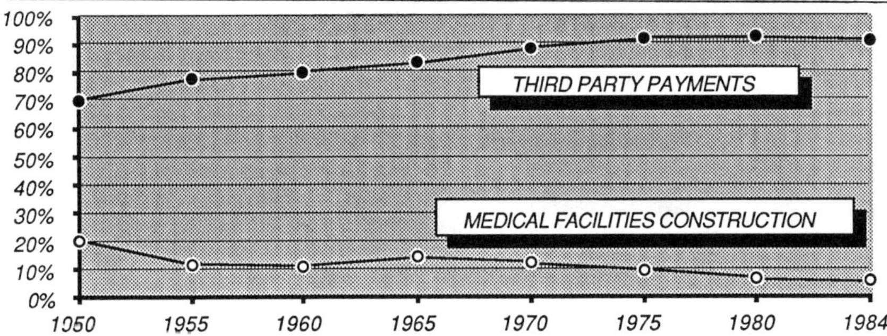

Source: Office of the Assistant Secretary for Planning and Evaluation, Department of Health and Human Services, *Hospital Capital Expenses: A Medicare Payment Strategy for the Future* (Washington, DC: Office of the Assistant Secretary, 1986).

historical-cost reimbursement: a decreased ability to make free-and-clear profits by keeping expenditures below revenues,[53] and the shortfall between depreciation payments based on historical cost and the actual replacement cost of buildings and equipment.

The Shift to Market Financing

As quasi-commercial enterprises, hospitals quickly turned to private capital markets and internal reserves (accumulated endowment and surplus earnings) to finance expansion, renovation, and expensive new technology (such as coronary and intensive care units, cardiac catheterization laboratories and open heart surgery programs, and radiation therapy). Exhibit 1-1 traces the growth of U.S. medical facility construction expenditures as a percentage of all U.S. hospital expenditures since 1950, and displays it alongside the growth in the percentage of hospital revenues received from third-party payers over this same period. Although construction costs and third-party payment both grew, often dramatically, during this period, the percentage of total hospital expenditures attributable to construction costs dropped steadily. This is because operating costs grew even more quickly than capital costs. Despite the massive increase in physical capital, there was no aggregate substitution of capital for other inputs in the production of care.

Once investment brokerage firms convinced state legislatures to establish bonding authorities that could issue tax-exempt debt on behalf of hospitals without requiring hospitals to pass ownership title to the state, access to capital increased even more dramatically.[54] Hospitals

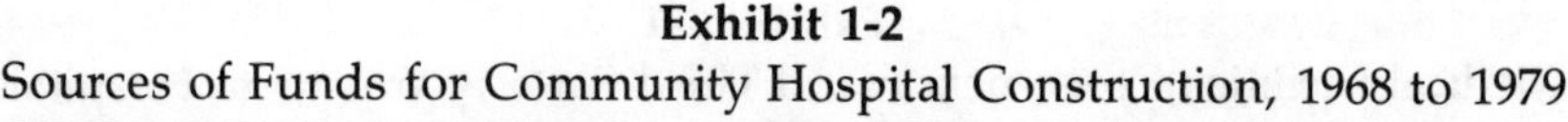
Exhibit 1-2
Sources of Funds for Community Hospital Construction, 1968 to 1979

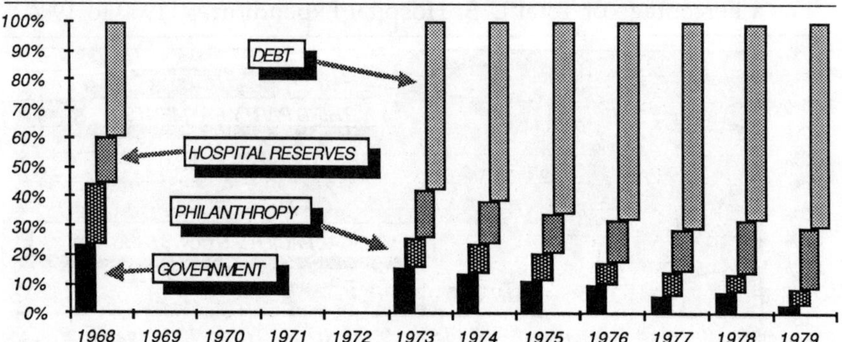

Source: Commission on Capital Policy, *Report of the Commission on Capital Policy* (Washington, DC: American Health Planning Association, 1984), p. 12.

took advantage of it. As measured in constant 1967 dollars, hospitals issued $216 million in tax-exempt revenue bonds in 1971, $1,215 million in 1975, $2,607 million in 1977, and $1,850 million in 1981.[55] They spent most of the funds they raised through revenue bonds on renovation and new construction. In 1978, the most recent year for which reliable nationwide data about the components of construction debt are available, hospitals raised fully 82 percent of all construction-related debt through tax-exempt bonds.[56]

Exhibit 1-2 graphically documents the increasing reliance on all forms of debt to finance construction. Debt sources grew from 39 percent of construction funding in 1968 to 71 percent in 1979. As indebtedness grew, the relative contributions of other construction funding sources receded. Between 1968 and 1979, the percent of construction costs met by governmental funds (including construction initiated by government-owned hospitals) fell from 23 percent to 16 percent, and the percent financed by philanthropy fell even more abruptly from 21 percent to 5 percent.[57]

The importance of tax-exempt debt lies not only in its rapid rise to dominance as a source of construction funding, but in the nature of the debt itself. Tax-exempt bonds are revenue bonds. Unlike mortgages, which give the lender the right to assume ownership of real property if the hospital defaults, revenue bonds pledge future operating profits and obligate the hospital to manage its operations to produce the promised profits. Lenders can bring in their own managers if the hospital's current managers fail to perform. Tax-exempt bonds are rated for sale on the basis of the predicted likelihood that the hospital can make sufficient profits to repay. Access to the tax-exempt market depends on a hospital's ability to demonstrate both the potential and the commitment to generate operating surpluses.

Part of this volume of debt represents refinancing of existing tax-exempt obligations. Refinancing became popular in part because hospitals could structure tax-exempt bond repayment schedules to load interest costs into the early years and defer principal payments. Cost-based payers like Medicare reimbursed for the full current cost of interest plus the straight-line average cost of depreciation: because depreciation reimbursement greatly exceeded principal payments in the early years, institutions received millions of dollars in early reimbursement. This surplus could be saved or spent, at the hospital's discretion, and if spent, hospitals could later refinance to postpone the large principal payments when these ultimately came due.[58] Medicare, commercial insurers, and most Blue Cross plans did not require hospitals to fund and earn interest on depreciation accounts in anticipation of these later payments (or of borrowing costs when fully depreciated assets had to be replaced).

As the tax-exempt market heated up and the nation's oversupply of beds continued to grow, Congress—whose budget was increasingly jeopardized by the war in Vietnam and by the rapid growth of hospital costs that excess beds helped induce—began to withdraw its support for public financing through the Hill-Burton program. Loans and loan guarantees were substituted for grants, and major funding cuts began in 1972. After 1975, no new funds were appropriated and all that remained of Hill-Burton was an agency to oversee outstanding grants and loans and help manage an off-budget mortgage insurance program. This program, popularly known as the "HUD 242 program," actually made considerable money for the government through the fees it charged. Although the large number of institutions in the government's insurance pool permitted the 242 program to be slightly less restrictive than private bond insurance firms, hospitals that could not gain access to debt markets on the strength of their own finances did not qualify for this insurance. For the roughly 50 percent of hospitals that could qualify in the early 1980s, the program served mainly to lower interest rates by improving bond ratings.

The repeal of Hill-Burton completed a fundamental shift from a public policy that regarded hospital capital as a public investment provided and to some extent controlled by public sources (whether governmental or philanthropic) to a policy that saw capital as the private property of any hospital that could accumulate it through commercial success—even if that success were paid for by government entitlement programs and state-chartered and subsidized Blue Cross plans. "The Public's Investment in Hospitals," as Rorem had titled his path-breaking 1930 book, was given over to a group of increasingly commercially oriented institutions. Capital funds in the future were to come almost exclusively from private capital markets.

The Transformation of Proprietary Hospitals

Bond markets were not the only private capital markets that Medicare allowed hospitals to enter. The proprietary sector, which had been in decline between 1929 and the explosive growth of private hospital insurance in the 1940s and 1950s, and which had been hampered since that time by exclusion from Hill-Burton and disfavor among areawide planning groups, suddenly became attractive to investors. Not only did the proprietaries receive all the benefits that Medicare and private insurance conferred on voluntary hospitals, but they received an explicit return on equity from Medicare, as well as something of a blank check to acquire other hospitals. The blank check resulted from the fact that, until Congress finally "closed the account" in 1985, the full price paid for acquisition of additional facilities—even if wildly inflated—qualified for reimbursement as depreciable expense, along with any associated interest. Until 1985, it was even possible to pyramid acquisitions within multilayered corporate shells to extract potentially enormous windfall profits from Medicare and other payers.

Under such circumstances, it must have been difficult not to make handsome profits, and the control of proprietary hospitals began to shift from physician entrepreneurs to publicly traded corporations which acquired many hospitals. The number of short-term, acute care hospitals owned by for-profit hospital chains rose from 6 percent of all hospitals in 1977 to 10 percent in 1982.[59] These corporations, many of which began as contract managers of public and voluntary hospitals, also began to acquire each other in a process of consolidation that attracted considerable attention in the late 1970s and early 1980s. The five largest chains (Hospital Corporation of America, Humana, American Medical International, National Medical Enterprises, and Lifemark) more than doubled their total beds between 1976 and 1981, to 62,820.[60] By 1987, however, a major spokesman and analyst of the proprietary hospital industry, Robert A. Vraciu, was explaining that "hospital acquisition has slowed to a trickle" and that Medicare reform and increased price competition throughout the system had begun to make the hospital business less of a sure thing.[61] By this time, several of the large hospital chains had begun to divest and restructure. Word reached the newspapers of a plan by Vraciu's own employer, the Hospital Corporation of America, to sell nearly half of its hospitals to a group of its own managers.

Exhibit 1-3 traces changes in the relative percentage of U.S. community hospital beds under proprietary, public, and voluntary owner-

while only 53 percent of single-facility offerings achieved this level of investor confidence.[82]

As the generous reimbursement environment of the late 1960s and the 1970s began to give way in the 1980s, the hope of better access to capital convinced many hospitals to sacrifice their autonomy and join for-profit or nonprofit multi-institutional alliances and systems.[83] Between 1975 and 1980, American Hospital Association data indicate that the number of U.S. multihospital systems grew from 202 to 256.[84] Some consolidation in the number of systems occurred in the early 1980s, but the number of hospitals and beds under multi-institutional control continued to grow. In 1975, one-quarter of U.S. community hospitals belonged to systems; by 1982, the proportion had reached one-third. Although the number of beds leased or owned by for-profit entities continued to grow at least through 1984,[85] nonprofit systems grew more quickly.[86] After 1982, as the reimbursement environment grew less permissive, systems resisted acquiring the financially weaker hospitals that appear to have constituted most of the remaining candidates for acquisition.[87] Stock prices of the for-profit chains also plummeted.[88] These organizations increasingly invested the considerable capital they had accumulated in nursing homes, mental hospitals, health maintenance organizations, nonhealth businesses, and foreign countries.[89]

In addition to joining large systems and alliances, many freestanding voluntary hospitals changed their legal structure to facilitate growth and diversification, often in partnership with private investors.[90] Until Congress changed the law in 1986, tax policy in the form of accelerated depreciation schedules for real estate enabled hospitals to form syndicates with private investors to build facilities like medical office buildings and ambulatory surgery centers without contributing any of their own capital. Under certain circumstances, tax policy also allowed nonprofit institutions to sell buildings, equipment, or land to private individuals and then lease it back.[91] This provided the institution with a one-time infusion of cash in return for a continuing lease payment obligation, and gave to the purchaser depreciation-related tax deductions that the nonprofit could not use.[92]

The effects of these tax provisions were fourfold. First, they helped better-off nonprofit hospitals raise capital to start ventures like ambulatory surgery centers, medical office buildings, and freestanding "urgicenters." Second, they presumably encouraged nonprofit institutions to emphasize ventures that were self-financing over other, less readily funded services and programs that may have had greater public health importance. Third, they encouraged hospitals to provide services under investor-owned rather than community-governed auspices. Fourth, these tax provisions encouraged hospitals to disaggregate their legal structure to accommodate the financing arrangements favored by tax policy.[93] A study of hospital corporate restructuring in Massachusetts conducted by the Health Capital Project revealed that a large percentage of freestanding, voluntary, acute care hospitals changed their legal structure in the early 1980s. In less regulated states, the incentives to restructure took hold earlier and even more strongly.[94]

The third major effect of relying on private capital is to give specifically for-profit organizations a great capital-raising advantage over nonprofits. For-profits not only enjoy an important extra source of capital—equity investors—but, unlike the principal of a loan, the purchase price of stock is rarely repaid by the issuing institution. (The promise of high future earnings or capital gains is necessary to maintain the value of stock once it has been sold, however.)

The sale of stock increases a company's ability to attract market capital by as much as tenfold or more, depending on such factors as the price-earnings ratio of the company's stock at the time of sale. In the middle 1980s, an A-rated voluntary hospital seeking to enter the tax-exempt bond market needed about $2.50 of profit or "surplus" projected forward through the life of a 30-year bond to secure about $15.00 of debt.[95] The investor-owned hospital could have used this same $2.50 to pay dividends on a new issue of stock. At a price-earnings ratio of 20:1—not uncommonly high during this period—this $2.50 stream of profit would have attracted $50.00 in new equity capital. This new equity, in turn, could be used to secure at least another $50.00 in debt because lenders to for-profit firms do not require the diversion of revenues to guarantee their bonds: they know that earnings to stockholders will be cut first if the borrower encounters any financial difficulty.[96] So, while the nonprofit hospital received $15.00 for its $2.50 stream of surplus, the for-profit firm could leverage $100.00. Of course, the investor-owned hospital would have to make additional profit on its $50.00 of debt to pay it back, together with profit to cover perhaps an additional $50.00 in interest.[97] Luckily for the hospital's investors, Medicare and most other payers reimbursed for the full cost of this principal and interest during this period. Medicare also provided automatic reimbursement to cover stock dividend payments at rates in the vicinity of 20 percent (!) when interest rates were high.[98] The fact that investor-owned hospitals must pay corporate income taxes appears not to have diluted significantly these capital-raising advantages.

The fourth major effect of private market capitalization during the 1967-to-1987 period was to cut off access to capital for organizations that could not create surpluses or profits. Such organizations cannot attract either debt or equity capital in their own right, and they are unattractive candidates for acquisition by multi-institutional systems. Unprofitable delivery institutions are not viable over the long term, and many closed. In New York City, for example, 35 hospitals totaling 4,586 beds closed between 1963 and 1977. Closures practically ceased after the enactment of Medicare and Medicaid in 1966, but they resumed again after New York's rate regulation program began to limit charges and revenues. Many of the hospitals that closed were small proprietaries and somewhat larger voluntaries that were left behind when their physicians moved their practices to the suburbs and their paying patients left their neighborhoods.[99] New York City was both greatly overbedded and highly regulated compared to other areas during this period, though, and its experience may not have been representative.

A more recent study by Mullner and McNeil found that 340 hospitals closed in the United States between 1980 and 1985, accounting for nearly 50,000 beds.[100] Rural hospitals had a lower rate of closure during this period than urban hospitals. Among community hospitals, small hospitals were much more likely to close; the six-year rate of closure reached 50 percent among urban community hospitals with fewer than 25 beds. At the county level, however, very few communities were left without a community hospital as a result of these closures. Other research suggests that, in the case of urban community hospitals, closure can be attributed primarily to the economic status of the neighborhoods and population groups served by financially distressed hospitals.[101] Thus, the policy of requiring private capitalization reduced access to hospital and emergency care for poor and minority populations.

The Structure of Health Care Financing

The behavior that resulted from treating nominally nonprofit hospitals like quasi-commercial enterprises and requiring them to acquire capital from private markets cannot be fully understood without reference to the underlying structure of health *care* (as distinct from health *capital*) financing in the United States prior to 1987. Health insurance in the United States was designed to accommodate fee-for-service medicine and the hospital system that grew up to serve private physicians. The practical demands of a financing system composed of independent intermediaries who reimburse providers without managing the production of services reinforced this initial emphasis on physician and hospital services. In such a system, covered services must be clearly defined, must be assigned a cost or price, and must be as free as possible of the "moral hazard" of uncontrollable discretionary utilization. Tests and treatments that require the use of drugs, supplies, equipment, and operative procedures are easily counted and hence more "insurable" than counseling, teaching, listening, and other less quantifiable activities.[102]

They also are services whose use can be limited to a single professional group to which entry barriers are high—physicians.

Because greater capital investment capacity accrues to services and institutions that are reimbursed by insurers, U.S. insurance mechanisms concentrated capital resources in acute care hospitals and, within hospitals, in facilities that supported more remunerative activities (such as surgery) and promoted a technology-intensive style of care. This insurance-based financing system produced a configuration of capital resources that is almost certainly not optimal given the health needs of the population.[103]

The predominantly private and fragmented structure of the health insurance system also generated financial pressures that denied some hospitals access to capital. Insurers, competing for the business of increasingly cost-conscious corporations and unions during the 1980s, sought to limit the revenues they paid out, in order to reduce premium costs. Major corporations, most of which were self-insured by the middle 1980s, also began to demand price reductions and to build copayments and utilization review provisions into the health insurance they offered their employees. (Government used similar measures to control its expenditures for Medicaid and, more recently, for Medicare.) Because a few of these payers in any given local area typically controlled large portions of the revenues health providers earned, they enjoyed monopsonistic power over provider institutions. This potentially allowed them to reduce their payments below levels capable of replenishing physical capital. (In classically competitive markets, by contrast, producers set prices high enough to meet capital needs.) In New York City, where hospitals have been under significant financial pressure for several years, more than half the voluntary hospitals could not meet the minimum criteria of bond-rating agencies by 1980, and the gap between the financially healthy and the financially unhealthy was widening.[108]

A further structural factor creating fiscal problems for health delivery institutions was the nonuniversal character of health insurance entitlement. Neither private carriers nor the federal government provided affordable insurance for many of the unemployed, for part-time workers, for employees of small firms, for rural residents, or for a sizable segment of the working poor.[105] This created a large pool of uninsured or self-insured patients, usually of very limited financial means, who were often unable to pay for medical services they might require. Additionally, state-managed Medicaid programs for the insured poor were parsimonious in their payments to hospitals. Together, these gaps in coverage, eligibility, and reimbursement created a situation in which delivery institutions that served the less well-off could not generate a sufficient surplus to attract private capital. Simultaneously, hospitals that enjoyed access to private capital rarely invested in areas where the payer mix was poor, or in services utilized primarily by the poor and uninsured.[106]

The race-, class-, and gender-related impacts of unequal access to capital are striking. In an analysis of zip codes in New York City in 1980, the Health Capital Project found that zip code areas dependent on voluntary hospitals without access to capital markets contained far more black, Hispanic, and poor residents and more female single-parent families than did the city as a whole.[107] Other research by Arthur Schatzkin and by Alan Sager supports these findings.[108]

Attempts at Corrective Regulation and Planning

Although reliance on private capital markets was the dominant capital policy during the 1967-to-1987 period, the enactment of Medicare also marked the beginning of federal efforts to impose regulatory restraints on health capital investment. It was not unlike the federal government's efforts to discourage smoking while subsidizing tobacco farming. The policy of relying on private markets as sources of capital interacted with historical-cost reimbursement, while employment-based entitlement stimulated overinvestment, selective underservice, and cost inflation. At the same time, planning and capital expenditure regulation tried to prevent these problems. In the years after Medicare, it became increasingly apparent how weak plan writing and capital regulation were in the face of strong economic incentives.

The first attempt at federally mandated planning and capital expenditure control was the comprehensive health planning (CHP) program. Enacted by Congress in 1968, CHP imposed an official end to the brief flowering of voluntary areawide planning in the United States. Critics had charged, in Anne Somers's words, that the voluntary planning movement

> set its sights too low for the urgency of the present situation. They claim that the voluntary planning movement has been too negative, with too much emphasis on saying "No" to unneeded facilities rather than on helping the hospitals develop needed facilities and services [Pittsburgh and Rochester may have been exceptions to the rule]; that it tends to favor minor needs, backed by money, rather than major needs, where money may be harder to find; that it has given too much attention to beds and too little to ambulatory and other facilities; that it has been too preoccupied with facilities at the expense of programs and services and with finances rather than professional relations; that it has tended to favor the *status quo*, and to discourage innovation and new entrants into the hospital field; that the councils are too heavily representative of the providers and not enough of consumers; and that most of them would not be viable without large-scale government financial support, which, almost by definition, contradicts the concept of "voluntarism."[109]

Congress stipulated that local comprehensive health planning agencies would be governed by community boards with consumer majorities, and it directed these agencies to plan all health-related activities in their region, from environmental health to primary care to tertiary services. Congress provided almost no carrots or sticks to help them accomplish this daunting task, however. Congress also provided very little in the way of operating funds or administrative guidance, although it did transfer to the CHP agencies the funds that voluntary areawide planning agencies had previously received. It required agencies to get the rest of their money from the very hospitals whose domination they were supposed to overturn. In sum, CHP agencies had little money, less federal guidance, and no regulatory power. In addition, they were saddled with a statutory requirement not to interfere with "existing patterns of private professional practice of medicine."[110]

Passed after little congressional debate, the new law reflected fundamental changes in the way Americans viewed community leadership and control. Grassroots civil rights struggles beginning in the 1950s challenged the right and ability of business, social, and political elites to define community needs. President Johnson's War on Poverty programs bypassed state and local government to give direct control of funds to beneficiary communities. "Maximum feasible participation" was the order of the day. Much more attention was paid to community health deficits, and rapid medical care cost inflation also attracted increasing concern. Because of the program's design, however, its principal outcome appears to have been a series of excruciating and lengthy turf battles enacted across the country, either between new CHP agencies and existing hospital councils, or within CHP boards. As one observer remarked at the time, "To the 'non-system' of health care that comprehensive health planning was intended to correct has been added a layer of 'non-planning' "[111]

Even before the enactment of CHP, some areawide planning leaders had begun to create governmental regulatory programs to review and approve hospital investment proposals. The movement began in New York in 1964, when that state's legislature enacted recommendations of a commission chaired by Rochester's Marion Folsom to set formulaic limits on hospital per diem cost reimbursement and create the nation's first certificate of need program. Folsom had grown discouraged with voluntary planning: he found that Rochester hospitals ignored community concerns once the pool of capital raised by his citywide fund drive had been spent. By 1968, there was a national drive for CoN laws, supported by the AHA and many state hospital associations. But such CoN programs were to prove relatively ineffectual in most areas, partly because it was easier for corporate leaders to limit their own donations than for state governments and provider-dominated planning boards to limit local spending of federal dollars.

Then, in 1972, Congress created the "1122 program," which required hospitals in participating states to receive planning approval for major capital expenditures or lose Medicare reimbursement for the investment. (Congress failed to pass a requirement that hospitals fund depreciation accounts, however.) With the enactment of the 1122 program, more and more states, prompted by rapid inflation in the cost of their Medicaid programs and disappointed by federal and industry inaction, established all-payer capital expenditure control programs and hospital rate-setting systems. By 1974, nearly half the states operated CoN programs.[112]

In 1975, Congress replaced the ineffective CHP program with the National Health Planning and Resources Development Act, P.L. 93-641, which mandated CoN in every state.

P.L. 93-641 established rules to determine which projects and services would be subject to CoN review and instructed the federal Department of Health and Human Services to promulgate national standards to guide state-level reviews. In addition, the law created over 200 health systems agencies (HSAs) to advise in the CoN process, and required the HSAs and 50 newly created state health planning and development agencies to write periodic master plans for health, supplemented by annual implementation plans. Congress did not enforce any consistency between plans and CoN decisions, though.

Complex rules for the composition of HSA and state agency governing boards were imposed in an attempt to guarantee political control by consumers and promote community rather than institutional health. States and HSAs created governing boards with consumer majorities, but their consumer members were not backed up by organized constituencies that cared enough about what planning agencies did to hold their supposed representatives accountable. Provider representatives, on the other hand, generally knew what their employers or their colleagues wanted and felt obliged to represent these preferences.[113] The governance rules created great political difficulties for agencies and added to their image as crude federal transplants into local political culture. More often than not, the rules failed to achieve their purpose: industry representatives with data and professional expertise still dominated governing boards, most of which failed to share the federal government's concern with cost control, in any event.

On the regulatory side, the focused interest of institutional applicants may have created even greater havoc: given the legalistic, standards-based nature of regulatory decision making and the typically low levels of funding and expertise of CoN agencies, applicants able to demand third-party reimbursement for any number of lawyers and consultants found it possible to "game" the regulations. They typically kept several steps ahead of procedural reforms.

Congressional appropriation of funds for the "planning law" at the time of passage fell well below what the committees designing the bill had authorized. Appropriations declined in subsequent years. Uncertain administration at HHS, together with congressional reluctance to strengthen the program's regulatory powers, enact national health insurance, or impose effective hospital rate controls, further crippled the law. Congress rejected a 1978 proposal by the Carter administration to establish capital pools. After years of survival by "continuing resolution" and declining financial support, Congress allowed the Health Planning and Resources Development Act to lapse on October 1, 1986. Most states continued their CoN programs, however, sometimes with higher thresholds for review.[114] Some states, including New York, Massachusetts, and Maine, also imposed or attempted to impose dollar limits on the total dollar impact of annual CoN approvals.[115] As of this writing, many HSAs survive with state and private sector support.

NOTES

Portions of this chapter take their inspiration from an article by Jonathan B. Brown and Richard Saltman, "Health Capital Policy in the United States: A Strategic Perspective," *Inquiry* 22 (Summer 1985): 122–33.

1. Jonathan B. Brown and Harry M. Marks, "Buying the Future: The Relationship between the Purchase of Physical Capital and Total Expenditure Growth in U.S. Hospitals." In *Health Capital Issues* (Washington, DC: Department of Health and Human Services, 1980), pp. 27–46.
2. C. Rufus Rorem, *The Public's Investment in Hospitals* (Chicago: University of Chicago Press, 1930), p. 30.
3. Ibid., p. 14.
4. Commission on Hospital Care, *Hospital Care in the United States* (New York: Commonwealth Fund, 1947).
5. Rorem, *The Public's Investment*, p. 210.
6. Ibid., p. 206.
7. Ibid., p. 184, 202.
8. Ibid., p. 218.
9. Ibid.
10. One of the reasons hospitals resisted this idea was their tradition of putting donors, often in great numbers, on their governing boards. Hospitals feared that the even larger numbers of donors to community chests would assume a governing role and disrupt the special relationships they enjoyed with particular donors and with religious and ethnic communities.
11. Daniel M. Fox, *Health Policies, Health Politics: The British and American Experience 1911–1965* (Princeton: Princeton University Press, 1986), p. 76.
12. Commission on Hospital Care, *Hospital Care*, pp. 531–33.

13. Hospital Survey of New York, *Report*, 3 vol. (New York: United Hospital Fund, 1938).
14. Herbert Klarman, "Planning for Facilities." In Eli Ginzberg, ed., *Regionalization and Policy*, DHEW publication no. (HRA) 77-623 (Washington, DC: U.S. Government Printing Office, 1977), p. 27.
15. Robert M. Sigmond and Thomas M. Tierney, "Could Capitation Ease Blue Cross Ills?" *Modern Hospital* (August 1965): 103–4.
16. Commission on Hospital Care, *Hospital Care*, p. 574.
17. Ibid., p. 567.
18. Ibid., p. 575.
19. Ibid., p. 550.
20. Commission on Hospital Care, *Hospital Care*.
21. Brian M. Kinkead, "Medicare Payment and Hospital Capital: The Evolution of Policy," *Health Affairs* 3 (1984): 49–74.
22. Klarman, "Planning for Facilities," p. 27.
23. Judith Lave and Lester Lave, *The Hospital Construction Act: An Evaluation of the Hill-Burton Program, 1948–1973* (Washington, DC: American Enterprise Institute for Public Policy Research, 1974).
24. Sylvia A. Law, *Blue Cross, What Went Wrong?* (New Haven: Yale University Press, 1974).
25. Bruce C. Vladeck, "America's Hospitals," *Health Affairs* 5 (1986): 100–107; Robert M. Sigmond, "Re-Examining the Role of the Community Hospital in a Competitive Environment," The Michael M. Davis Lecture, Center for Health Administration Studies, University of Chicago, 1985.
26. There were exceptions. The Michigan Blue Cross plan and a few other plans threatened to refuse to pay for excessive capital investment in the 1960s. The Kansas City plan lost an antitrust suit after it denied reimbursement to a hospital built over the objections of the local planning agency during the late 1970s.
27. Office of the Assistant Secretary for Planning and Evaluation, Department of Health and Human Services, *Hospital Capital Expenses: A Medicare Payment Strategy for the Future* (Washington, DC: Office of the Assistant Secretary, 1986), p. 12.
28. J.L. Stambaugh, "A Study of the Sources of Capital Funds for Hospital Construction in the United States," *Inquiry* 14 (1967): 14.
29. Ibid. Church-sponsored hospitals apparently enjoyed better credit because the church's nonhospital assets could be pledged.
30. Kinkead, "Medicare Payment and Hospital Capital."
31. Ibid. Fifteen years of Hill-Burton funding had satisfied much of the rural need for hospital beds and, in 1962, the Hill-Burton bed need formula for hospitals was changed in ways that decreased planning constraints and favored growing suburban areas. In 1964, Congress doubled Hill-Burton appropriations and opened the door to support of modernization and renovation projects in addition to new construction.
32. For an unrealistic but nevertheless informative account of the Rochester experience, see Henry B. Makover and Leonard S. Rosenfield, *The Rochester Regional Hospital Council* (Cambridge, MA: Harvard University Press, 1956).
33. From its inception in 1946, Hill-Burton had effectively required community philanthropic support for the projects it funded. It did so by limiting the federal share of project expenses in most cases to less than 67 percent, and

by simultaneously limiting to 33 percent the maximum share that hospitals could finance through indebtedness. However, until the 1964 "Hill-Harris" amendments, the program did little to encourage state agencies to involve communities in planning. The amendments provided limited funds for community hospital councils but stopped short of giving them any voice or right of participation in the preparation of state annual facility plans, the documents that determined how Hill-Burton funds would be spent.

34. Herbert E. Klarman, "Economic Factors in Hospital Planning in Urban Areas," *Public Health Reports* 82 (1967): 726.
35. Regarding the replacement for the troubled proprietary hospital, Robert M. Sigmond was to remark in his 1985 Michael M. Davis lecture, "Re-Examining the Role," "I urge you to visit some of our most outstanding community hospitals, as Paul Starr and I did the other day at the Park Ridge Hospital in Rochester, New York, and study its transformation."
36. Dena Puskin, "The Birth of Regional Health Planning in the Rochester Region: 1960–1969," unpublished paper, November 1972.
37. Robert M. Sigmond, "A Practical Approach to Area-Wide Hospital Planning," *Hospital Administration in Canada* (July 1967): 24.
38. By 1964, a number of hospitals had obtained substantial funds for capital projects without official review by the association, and one hospital had gone ahead with a project after a negative review. Robert M. Sigmond, "Hospital Planning in Allegheny County," *Group Practice* 13 (June 1964): 370–74.
39. Steven Sieverts, "Book Review," *Health Services Research* (Fall 1968): 251–56, quoted in Anne R. Somers, *Hospital Regulation: The Dilemma of Public Policy* (Princeton: Industrial Relations Section, Princeton University, 1969).
40. William R. Foyle, "Accounting and Finance. Summary and Recommendations." In *Hospital and Medical Economics,* Walter J. McNerny, study director (Chicago: Hospital Research and Educational Trust, 1962), p. 998.
41. William R. Foyle, "Capital Funds and Depreciation and Replacement Costs." In *Hospital and Medical Economics,* Walter J. McNerny, study director (Chicago: Hospital Research and Educational Trust, 1962), p. 1000.
42. Robert M. Sigmond, "Hospital Capital Funds: Changing Needs and Sources," *Hospitals* (August 16, 1965): 52–55.
43. Robert M. Sigmond, "Depreciation as a Source of Capital Financing." In *Capital Financing of Hospitals—Sources and Concerns. A Report of the 1967 National Forum on Hospital and Health Affairs* (Chapel Hill, NC: Graduate Program in Hospital Administration, Duke University, no date), pp. 77–85.
44. Ibid., p. 82.
45. Anne R. Somers, *Hospital Regulation: The Dilemma of Public Policy* (Princeton: Industrial Relations Section, Princeton University, 1969), p. 138.
46. Ibid., p. 138.
47. Walter J. McNerny, in Lewis E. Weeks and Howard J. Berman, eds., *Shapers of American Health Policy: An Oral History* (Ann Arbor, MI: Health Administration Press, 1985), p. 178.
48. American Hospital Association, "Research Capsule No. 5," *Hospitals* 46 (March 1, 1972): 146; and "Research Capsule No. 17," *Hospitals* 49 (July 1, 1975): 83.
49. Office of the Assistant Secretary, *Hospital Capital Expenses,* p. 3.
50. Sigmond, "Hospital Capital Funds."

51. See Herman M. Somers and Anne R. Somers, *Medicare and the Hospitals: Issues and Prospects* (Washington, DC: Brookings Institution, 1967); Judith M. Feder, *Medicare: The Politics of Federal Hospital Insurance* (Lexington, MA: Lexington Books, 1977); Kinkead, "Medicare Payment and Hospital Capital"; Theodore R. Marmor, *The Politics of Medicare* (Hawthorne, NY: Aldine Publishing Co., 1973); Rashi Fein, *Medical Care, Medical Costs: The Search for a Health Insurance Policy* (Cambridge, MA: Harvard University Press, 1986).
52. Political concessions resulted in a number of additional capital-related bonuses. The government allowed hospitals to receive depreciation payments for assets already acquired and previously depreciated, and to do so according to an accelerated rather than a straight-line schedule. (Accelerated depreciation was later repealed.) Hospitals were not actually required to fund their depreciation accounts, however. A "plus factor" of 2 percent of allowable costs also was granted, apparently to satisfy hospital demands for recognition of the opportunity cost of invested equity capital – the profit hospitals could have earned had they invested their money outside the hospital. This sweetener was eliminated in 1969, "only to reemerge in the guise of a 'nursing differential,' " says Brian M. Kinkead in "Medicare Payment and Hospital Capital," p. 54.
53. Ray E. Brown, "Capital Financing: Origins and Dimensions of the Current Dilemma," *Journal of the American Hospital Association* 42 (October 16, 1968): 43–47, 112.
54. As compared to taxable bonds and commercial (bank) loans, the tax-exempt market offered hospitals much longer repayment periods, more flexible terms, 0 to 20 percent rather than 50 percent equity contribution requirements, lower interest rates, and access to a larger and more receptive group of potential buyers. For a good summary of these advantages see Kinkead, "Medicare Payment and Hospital Capital."
55. Anthony J. Taddey and Gordon Gayer, "Uses and Effects of Hospital Tax-Exempt Financing," *Hospital Financial Management* (July 1982): 10–30.
56. The primary sources for these data are surveys conducted by the American Hospital Association. Discussions with the AHA indicate that many hospitals probably gave imprecise answers; municipal and other hospitals that receive construction funds from governmental owners often do not know or do not report the ultimate source of their funds, for example, and the same problem arises with hospitals owned by multihospital systems. The questionnaire also did not distinguish between equity investment and retained earnings as sources of internal reserves. The fact that internal reserves began to recover as a source of funding in the late 1970s may reflect the increasing role of investor equity. Note also that the number of hospitals responding to the AHA surveys from year to year varied between 677 and 1,071; statistical corrections have been made to account for nonresponse (see Ross Mullner et al., "Funding Aspects of Construction in U.S. Hospitals (1973–1979)," *Hospital Financial Management* [November 1981]: 30–34), but the success of these calculations remains unknown. Rough comparisons of the total dollar volume of tax-exempt debt implied by the AHA's corrected data to actual tax-exempt borrowing appear to indicate some degree of residual undercounting.

Although the AHA conducted other construction funding surveys in 1981, 1983, and 1984, the questions and analyses are not comparable to the data reported in Exhibit 1-2 and changed from year to year. Consequently, I do not report the findings. It is clear that borrowing continued to grow after 1979, however. A combination of factors (including favorable interest rates, investment by hospitals in alternative delivery systems, and the desire to go to market before Congress restricted access to tax-exempt debt and repealed cost-based capital reimbursement) stimulated hospitals to sell nearly $22 billion in bonds in 1985, exclusive of refinancing issues (see Office of the Assistant Secretary, *Hospital Capital Expenses*). This amount doubles the previous annual record, set in 1982.

57. Taddey and Gayer, "Uses and Effects of Hospital Tax-Exempt Financing," p. 12.
58. Arthur Henkel, "Payment Policy Effects on Investor Behavior and Access to Capital." In *Health Capital Commission, Report of the Commission on Capital Policy* (Washington, DC: American Health Planning Association, 1984), pp. 80–87.
59. Bradford H. Gray, "An Introduction to the New Health Care for Profit." In Bradford H. Gray, ed., *The New Health Care for Profit: Doctors and Hospitals in a Competitive Environment* (Washington, DC: National Academy Press, 1983).
60. Richard B. Siegrist, "Wall Street and the For-Profit Hospital Management Companies." In Bradford H. Gray, ed., *The New Health Care for Profit: Doctors and Hospitals in a Competitive Environment* (Washington, DC: National Academy Press, 1983).
61. Robert A. Vraciu, "That Was Then, This Is Now," *Frontiers of Health Services Management* 3 (May 1987): 23–25.
62. Kinkead, "Medicare Payment and Hospital Capital" p. 58.
63. Ibid., p. 59.
64. Alan Sager, "Why Urban Voluntary Hospitals Close," *Health Services Research* 18 (Fall 1983): 451–57.
65. J.B. Silvers, "The Impact of Financial Policy and Structure on Investments in Health Care." In Gerald E. Bisbee and Robert A. Vraciu, eds., *Managing the Finances of Health Care Organizations* (Ann Arbor, MI: Health Administration Press, 1980), pp. 431–45.
66. M. Shain and M.I. Roemer, "Hospital Costs Related to the Supply of Beds," *Modern Hospital* 92 (1959): 73; M.I. Roemer and M. Shain, *Hospital Utilization under Insurance* (Chicago: American Hospital Association, 1959).
67. D. Harris, "An Elaboration of the Relationship between General Hospital Bed Supply and General Hospital Utilization," *Journal of Health and Social Behavior* 15 (1975): 162–72; J. May, "Utilization of Health Services and the Availability of Resources." In R. Anderson, ed., *Equity in Health Services* (Cambridge, MA: Ballinger, 1975); J. Rafferty, "Patterns of Hospital Use," *Journal of Political Economy* (1971): 154–65.
68. Brown and Marks, "Buying the Future."
69. Jonathan Brown and Marc J. Roberts, *Health Care Expenditures since 1950,* (Boston: School of Public Health, Harvard University, 1978).
70. Fein, *Medical Care, Medical Costs*.
71. Strictly speaking, much of this noncovered expenditure is not out-of-pocket because elders buy supplementary insurance from Blue Cross and other carriers.
72. James A. Morone and Andrew Dunham, "The Waning of Professional Dominance: DRGs and the Hospitals," *Health Affairs* 3 (1984): 85.

73. See Office of the Assistant Secretary, *Hospital Capital Expenses.*
74. Glenn Wilson, Cecil G. Sheps, and Thomas R. Oliver, "Effects of Hospital Revenue Bonds on Hospital Planning and Operations," *New England Journal of Medicine* 307 (1982): 1426–30.
75. Siegrist, "Wall Street."
76. Compensation for nonowning managers also often depends on profit performance. For a good review of the financial environment and activities of the for-profit hospital chains, see Siegrist, "Wall Street."
77. To be marketable, virtually all bond issuances must be rated for risk of default by one or both of the two major bond-rating organizations, Moody's and Standard and Poor's. Highly rated bonds are termed "investment grade," which implies a very low level of risk. The higher the rating, the lower the interest rate the hospital must pay to attract buyers, and the larger the market for its bonds.
78. See William O. Cleverley, *Hospital Industry Analysis Report,* Fifth Edition (Oak Brook, IL: Financial Analysis Service, Healthcare Financial Management Association, 1985).
79. Dan Ermann and John Gabel, "Multihospital Systems: Issues and Empirical Findings," *Health Affairs* 3 (1984): 50–64; Ernest W. Saward and E.K. Gallagher, "Reflections on Change in Medical Practice: The Current Trend to Large-Scale Medical Organization," *Journal of the American Medical Association* 250 (1983): 2820–25; American Hospital Association Advisory Panel on Capital, *Historical Linkages between Selected Hospital Characteristics and Bond Ratings* (Washington, DC: American Hospital Association, 1982).
80. D. Leigh Yanish, "Pooled Assets Expand Debt Capacity," *Modern Healthcare* 11 (October 1981): 86–88.
81. Michael Hernandez and C.G. Howie, "Capital Financing by Multihospital Systems." In Scott A. Mason, ed., *Multihospital Arrangements: Public Policy Implications* (Chicago: American Hospital Association, 1979), pp. 37–47.
82. Ermann and Gabel, "Multihospital Systems."
83. Alliances are joint ventures and other relationships that hospitals can join without sacrificing their legal autonomy. Systems comprise hospitals that are "leased, under contract management, legally incorporated, or under the direction of a board that determines the central direction of two or more hospitals." Ibid., p. 51.
84. Ibid.
85. Kenneth S. Abramowitz, *The Future of Health Care Delivery in America* (New York: Sanford C. Bernstein & Co., 1985); Myk Cherskov, "What's Driving Upcoming Mergers," *Hospitals* (January 5, 1987): 36–40.
86. Ermann and Gabel, "Multihospital Systems."
87. Jeffrey A. Alexander, Bonnie L. Lewis, and Michael A. Morrisey, "Acquisition Strategies of Multihospital Systems," *Health Affairs* 4 (1985): 49–66.
88. Stephen Wood, "Industry Notes," *Hospital Capital Finance* 3 (1986): 5.
89. Ermann and Gabel, "Multihospital Systems."
90. Ernst & Whinney, *Corporate Reorganization* (New York: Ernst & Whinney, 1984).
91. Siegrist, "Wall Street."
92. Congress restricted these "sale and lease back" arrangements to new technology in 1984, however.
93. Lawrence Gerber, *Hospital Restructuring: Why, When and How* (Chicago: Pluribus Press, 1983).

94. Ernst & Whinney, *Corporate Reorganization*.
95. This calculation assumes a "coverage ratio" requirement of 2.5—a $2.50 stream of earnings to cover an annual debt service payment of $1.00—and interest rates such that 50 percent of the hospital's debt service would repay interest by the time the bond was retired in 30 years. Thus, the amount borrowed equals $0.50 × 30 years.
96. This example assumes that lenders require a 50 percent debt-to-equity ratio in the for-profit firm. At one time during the early 1980s, the Hospital Corporation of America's debt-equity ratio reached 80 percent, and its price-earnings ratio exceeded 40:1. Extraordinary numbers like these imply a firm whose revenues are guaranteed by government but whose speculative investors expect to make a lot of money when its stock price rises.
97. In the taxable bond market, which lends money for shorter periods than the tax-exempt market, an additional profit stream of $5.00 per year would be required to retire this debt in 20 years, necessitating a before-tax return on investment of about 10 percent, roughly equivalent to the after-tax price-earnings ratio of 20:1 assumed in this example.
98. In the Medicare law, the rate of reimbursement for return on equity was set at 1.5 times the interest paid on debt issued by the Medicare trust fund.
99. Karen M. Pleines, "Hospital Closures: The New York City Experience." In *Hospital Closures in New York City* (New York: United Hospital Fund of New York, 1980), pp. 16–39.
100. Russ M. Mullner and David McNeil, "Urban and Rural Hospital Closures," *Health Affairs* 5 (Fall 1986): 131–41.
101. Judith M. Feder and Jack Hadley, *Cutbacks, Recession and Care to the Poor: Will the Urban Poor Get Hospital Care?* (Washington, DC: Urban Institute, 1983); Arthur Schatzkin, "The Relationship of Inpatient Racial Composition and Hospital Closure in New York City," *Medical Care* 23 (1984): 379–87; Sager, "Why Urban Voluntary Hospitals Close"; Nancy M. Kane, "New York City Hospitals: Relationships among Hospital Financial Status, Claimed Capital Need, Likely Capital Access, and Community Characteristics," Health Capital Project Working Paper #6 (Boston: School of Public Health, Harvard University, 1984).
102. Eli Ginzberg, "The Monetarization of Medical Care," *New England Journal of Medicine* 310 (1984): 1162–65.
103. Institute of Medicine, *Controlling the Supply of Hospital Beds* (Washington DC: National Academy Press, 1976); Vladeck "America's Hospitals," p. 106.
104. Nancy M. Kane, "The Demise of Robin Hood: Implications for the Social Missions of Hospitals," Health Capital Project Working Paper #16 (Boston: School of Public Health, Harvard University, 1985).
105. S.E. Berki, Leon Wyszewianski, Richard Lichtenstein, et al., "Health Insurance Coverage of the Unemployed," *Medical Care* 23 (1985): 847–54; Karen Davis and Diane Rowland, "Uninsured and Underserved: Inequities in Health Care in the United States," *Milbank Memorial Fund Quarterly/Health and Society* 61 (1983): 149–76.
106. Ekaterina Siafaca, *Investor-Owned Hospitals and Their Role in the Changing U.S. Health Care System* (New York: F & S Press, 1981), pp. 83–117.
107. Kane, *New York City Hospitals*.
108. Schatzkin, "The Relationship"; Sager, "Why Urban Voluntary Hospitals Close."

109. Somers, *Hospital Regulation*, p. 140.
110. Public Law 89-749, Comprehensive Health Planning Act, preamble.
111. Bonnie Lefcowitz, *Health Planning: Lessons for the Future* (Rockville, MD: Aspen Systems Corporation, 1983), p. 13.
112. Ibid.
113. Theodore R. Marmor and James A. Morone, "Representing Consumer Interests: Imbalanced Markets, Health Planning, and the HSAs," *Milbank Memorial Fund Quarterly* 58 (1980): 125–65; Bruce Vladeck, "Interest Group Representation and the HSAs: Health Planning and Political Theory," *American Journal of Public Health* 67 (1977): 23–29.
114. James B. Simpson, "State Certificate of Need Programs: The Current Status," *American Journal of Public Health* 75 (1985): 1225–29.
115. Wendy M. Greenfield, "New Approaches to Using the Determination of Need Process to Contain Hospital Costs," *New England Journal of Medicine* 309 (1983): 372–74; Carol V. Getts, *Methods for Establishing Capital Expenditure Limits* (Madison, WI: Institute for Health Planning, 1984); ICF, Inc., *An Analysis of Programs to Limit Hospital Expenditures. Final Report.* (Washington, DC: ICF, Inc., 1980).

2.

Health Capital Policy in the Future

1988–2000: HOSPITALS LEAVE CENTER STAGE

Hospitals dominated the health care delivery system in the United States between the end of World War II and the mid-1980s. Physician preferences drove their administrative decision making and competitive planning throughout this period, and a greater share of the nation's health care dollar went to acute care hospitals than to any other class of health care organization or health professional group. Hospitals accumulated an even greater share of the nation's health capital investment. Their ability to prosper and accumulate capital depended on geographic location or a willingness to avoid admitting patients not covered by private insurance or government entitlement, however; the wealth dispensed to hospitals fell unevenly. By 1987, the most salient distinction among general hospitals was the distinction between wealthy hospitals and poor hospitals, between hospitals serving well-to-do communities or groups and hospitals that serve a much greater share of the poor.[1]

Although we hear much rhetoric about the virtues[2] and evils[3] of proprietary, voluntary, and public hospitals, the great majority of hospitals today would have to be considered primarily commercial in orientation. Indeed, many health policy analysts take this commercial orientation for granted. They assume that the plight of voluntary and public hospitals in poor urban neighborhoods results more from poor management—a failure to move to the suburbs while the getting was good, for example—than from social commitment or charity. The plight of troubled hospitals in rural areas, the same experts say, results from their small size (inherent economic inefficiency) and the lack of markets large enough to support them—not from any struggle to bring quality medical care to the hinterlands.

Despite their 40-year hegemony, their commercialism, and their accumulated wealth, independent community hospitals as we have known them are about to abandon center stage. They are victims—willing victims perhaps, but victims, nonetheless—of the fundamental miscalculation of postwar U.S. health financing policy, the idea that the nation could wash away the structural problems of its health care system by pouring tides of money into existing institutions. For most of the postwar period it has been politically easier to tax the populace and increase insurance premiums than to create institutions capable of controlling costs, easier to try to pay for indigent care with cost shifting (or by tolerating ill health for a minority of the population) than to confront the economic interests arrayed in opposition to publicly financed universal entitlement to health care. It has been easier to buy the appearance of quality care and access in the form of expensive technological marvels than to monitor hospital and physician practice seriously and report the results. It has been easier to build up an enormous investment in attempted curing than to step on economic toes to prevent disease. It has been easier to pretend that "community hospitals" could and would take responsibility for community health and for individual health maintenance than to create institutions specifically designed and managed for that purpose.

It appears that the nation can no longer afford the costs of its postwar strategy. The nation's international economic position is weakening, a huge federal deficit must be whittled down, Medicaid expenditures represent the largest single public expenditure in many state budgets, and business has awakened to the advantages it can reap by paying less for health insurance and maintaining a healthier work force. At the same time, the rapidly growing supply of physicians makes it far more difficult than it used to be for doctors to preserve the status quo; in fact, physicians in many areas are rushing to get in on the ground floor with a variety of organizations whose ultimate success lies in their ability to dictate physicians' terms of employment and control their professional behavior.

Hospitals, in the meantime, have come to the end of their long capital string. Originally financed by donations and government grants, hospitals starting in the 1960s leveraged their rise to commercial hegemony by pledging their newly found political strength and future revenues to secure debt. By the 1980s, the hospital industry had assumed a burden of long-term debt that was much larger, compared to total assets, than that of most other American industries. To finance further commercialization and growth in the 1970s and early 1980s, part of the industry turned to equity investors, who hoped for even greater commercial returns than did the lenders. The crash began in 1984 as Congress finally acted to eliminate cost-based reimbursement in the Medicare program, and business purchasers of health insurance demanded serious cost controls. Although hospitals on average increased their profits initially when Medicare's prospective payment system was introduced, bond-rating agencies began to raise the ante for investment-grade ratings. Proprietary hospitals chains performed worse during a historic bull market than did any other industry group save domestic oil producers (who suffered the effects of a drastic fall in the world price of oil).[4] Now, commercially oriented hospitals and hospital chains are turning to new lines of business, some health-related and some not, some in their own communities and some not even in their own nation, to preserve their independence and finance further growth. The market has not yet spoken its final word about the success of these enterprises, although in 1986 for-profit hospital chains began to abandon many of their new ventures, and businesses spun off by independent voluntary hospitals were said to be failing or losing money at a rapid rate (as new business ventures typically do throughout the economy). In 1987, the Hospital Corporation of America was negotiating to sell roughly half its hospitals. For the first time in a long time, one began to hear serious talk about a need to increase philanthropy[5] and about the political dangers of abandoning the hospital's traditional missions of community service and charity.[6]

The main locus of economic competition seems to be shifting from the provision of specific services, such as acute hospital care, to the development and sale to employers of care management products produced by good-sized regional and national firms.[7] These product lines will include all or some of the following care management models: staff- and group-model HMOs, network HMOs, independent practice associations (IPAs), preferred provider organizations (PPOs), and more traditional insurance plans backed up by utilization review and pretreatment certification. All these products are becoming less community-rated and more experience-rated, creating growing problems for a variety of groups, including employees of small firms and sufferers of chronic disease. It also seems likely that the insurance, HMO, hospital, and private practice sectors will continue to merge and consolidate, often into large regional and national care management corporations. These multidivisional corporations, organized for the most part on a for-profit basis, will be able to offer employers a range of care management models.[8] Such multioption firms may have an advantage over single-option organizations because they can free employers who use them from the difficult task of selecting and monitoring a variety of health insurance and health maintenance plans for their employees.

Brokering and management firms will assume some of the health planning responsibility that community and governmental organizations previously tried to carry out, including efforts to coordinate services and foster continuity of care. These multiproduct firms also will help balance investment across provider sectors, taking capital out of acute care and shifting it into long-term care and ambulatory care—and also into marketing, advertising, bureaucracy, and the pockets of investors and corporate parents. The shift of capital into long-term care will accelerate as life-care communities and long-term care insurance products are created and marketed to well-to-do purchasers.[9]

The Future for Hospitals

Hospitals will compete with each other for contracts with these care management systems, rather than competing primarily for physicians as they have in the past. Their competitive success will depend a great deal—although not entirely[10]—on the price at which they are able to provide care. Together with continuing unilateral reductions in the prices government is willing to pay, the oligopsonistic price pressure imposed by care management corporations will combine with widespread overbedding to make commercial success more and more difficult to achieve. Traditional sources of open-ended reimbursement, Blue Cross and commercial insurers, will shrink dramatically as these sources confront competition from managed care: these payers will either lose business to managed care, cease to offer open-ended reimbursement by demanding significant price discounts from hospitals, or become care managers themselves. Even if a sizable proportion of Americans ultimately reject the cost and coverage advantages of managed care and continue to purchase traditional insurance, the firms that sell traditional insurance will try to send their business to lower-cost hospitals in order to meet price competition in their industry.

To gain access to new capital and to repay existing debt, hospitals must somehow find ways to extract surpluses from declining revenues, or else increase revenues with higher utilization or new products. Higher utilization cannot provide a solution for the hospital industry as a whole, however, and new products themselves require new capital to launch.

Most hospitals also will find it difficult to tap the newest source of outside capital—the individual and corporate investors who see a bright future for HMOs and other producers of "managed care." This is because most hospitals are not organized physically, technically, socially, or economically to produce managed care. Hospitals were developed to provide workshops to private, fee-for-service physicians. Hospitals sell medical services of a certain kind, not insurance and not health maintenance. Although a few independent hospitals and some hospital chains have started HMO subsidiaries, most independent hospitals choose to diversify into other medical service "commodities" such as home care, ambulatory surgery, and fee-for-service primary care.[11]

Philanthropic contributions to voluntary hospitals and tax support of public hospitals may increase as the financial difficulties of these institutions attract attention. Even the most community-oriented voluntary hospital boards will find it difficult to maintain commitments to free care, emergency care, and public health programs, however. As a result, fewer and fewer hospitals are likely to fund their depreciation accounts fully; as most did in the years before Medicare and Medicaid, many will choose to spend revenues on current needs (including free care and other charitable and social responsibilities) rather than on savings or large capital projects. In the long run, absent concerted community or governmental intervention, the nation's hospital infrastructure may deteriorate both technically and structurally. Patient dumping and other reductions in community service and quality of care may also continue to spread.

The voluntary hospitals that can meet community commitments will be located, for the most part, in the well-to-do communities that least need the community services and the charity. The pattern of hospital closures in poor urban neighborhoods and rural areas that goes back to at least the 1960s will continue if not accelerate. It is possible that many communities will lose their "sole community provider" hospital if government does not act. Quality of care in and access to both ambulatory and hospital services are likely to deteriorate, perhaps catastrophically in some areas.

The question of what public action may be taken in response to infrastructure decay, hospital closure, dumping, and related problems will determine not only the magnitude of these problems but the longer-run trajectory of system change. Congress is currently considering legislation to establish federal catastrophic health insurance and federalize management of the Medicaid program. Many states may continue, and others may initiate free care and bad debt pools to support indigent care in hospitals and health centers. Some states may organize these pools on a modified voucher basis to promote competition and increase institutional responsiveness to beneficiary needs. Proprietary and not-for-profit HMOs will not step forward to locate and market services to beneficiaries in unprofitable low-income areas, however, so that planning, construction, and working capital funds to create HMOs in underserved areas may be needed. There will be pressure also to subsidize the capital needs of hospitals that provide essential services to isolated communities or to disadvantaged community groups. As a variety of cost-effective health services that cannot profitably be sold through the care management market disappear, or fail to be offered, governmental and philanthropic efforts to provide them will be proposed. Many hospitals may try to return to philanthropy as a source of significant financing for both capital and operating needs. To attract philanthropy, at least some hospitals will attend more seriously to community needs and yield greater control over their operations to community representatives. A geometrically expanding epidemic of acquired immune deficiency syndrome (AIDS) could catalyze both a renewed commitment of public resources and a reassertion of community and governmental authority.

New Capital Payment Policies: Market Payment versus Planned Payment

The question of how governments and communities will respond to the problems and opportunities of the new competition is a question about the relative roles of markets versus political and community institutions. In specific policy debates—whether and how to protect the health of the uninsured, for example—the question is often posed in either-or terms: markets versus planning and negotiation, markets versus regulation, markets versus public management. In the larger picture, however, governmental and community responses should eventually establish a new division of labor between markets and politics, and (with luck) create markets and political arrangements that reinforce and facilitate each other.

The repeal of cost-based reimbursement for hospital capital expenditures represents one episode in this evolving division of labor, one brushstroke on the larger canvas. Continued reliance on cost-based capital reimbursement no longer offers a viable option for most payers. To replace cost-based reimbursement, payers can imitate commercial markets either by eliminating explicit capital payments altogether or by building a formulaic capital allowance into prospective payments for operating costs; alternatively, they can create independent political institutions to receive and allocate capital funds on the basis of community-wide plans and priorities. We call these models *market payment* and *planned payment*, respectively.

Planned payment differs from market payment and cost-based reimbursement of capital in fundamental respects. Whereas cost-based and market payment create institutional entitlements, leave investment decision making primarily to institutions, and govern allocation with rules that for the most part ignore local circumstances and priorities, planned payment systems operate more like the head office of a decentralized multidivisional corporation. Large private corporations allocate limited corporate capital based on evaluations of divisional proposals and negotiations with and among division executives. Both the merits of specific divisional proposals and the overall structure and strategy of the larger entity are considered during the negotiation-allocation process.[15] The hospital fund drive led by Marion Folsom in Rochester (described in Chapter 1) and the Hill-Burton program represent forms of planned payment.

Subsequent sections of this chapter mainly explore the likely consequences of exclusive use of market payment. Of course, market payment and planned payment are far from mutually exclusive. Each probably works best in the presence of the other. Still, it aids the mental digestion to start with a clear understanding of how market payment would work in isolation. Many of its consequences are adverse. The worst cry out for nonmarket correction. The chapter therefore closes with an initial formulation of a planned payment structure that could remedy market payment's side-effects while retaining its benefits.

Although capital payment policy is just one color on the canvas, the conflict between market and planned capital payment illuminates much that is important in the big picture of future health system development and policy. Three things make a focused evaluation of capital policies so interesting.

First, the conflict between market and planned structures is common to most if not all of the health policy choices we now face. In the aggregate, these choices constitute the larger environment that will drive future health capital behavior (as well as—on the operating side—access, quality, and productivity). A detailed analysis of the market vs. planning choice in one particular policy area lends concreteness to what is often an overly abstract and ideological debate.

Second, the institutional proposal that emerges from this focused analysis provides a foundation on which nonmarket activity in several areas besides hospital capital payment could be built. In fact, it will emerge that a successful planned capital payment institution probably requires some control of both capital and operating funds as well as a diversified portfolio of policy responsibilities. Thus, the analysis ends up with a much broader relevance than its starting point might suggest.

Third, the rules by which third-party payers reimburse hospitals for capital needs and expenses are themselves important, not only to health capital behavior but to the larger goals of access, quality, and efficiency. It is true that the percentage of hospital revenues represented by capital reimbursement is small—5 percent to 10 percent—and that payers in the United States have rarely required hospitals to devote reimbursement for past capital expenditures to future capital purposes. Nevertheless, in reasonably well-off communities, cost-based reimbursement for depreciation and interest has strongly affected capital investment by partially insulating investment funds from depredation by the larger economic environment. In recent decades, some form of capital reimbursement independent of operating revenues was absolutely essential to continued capital investment.

At least in theory, a separate mechanism for capital reimbursement is less essential in the more open competitive health services market that seems to be emerging. Economically successful hospitals will have more freedom to make profits from operations and can use these profits to finance investment and borrowing and to attract equity investors. *Freedom* to make profits does not necessarily imply *ability* to make profits, however. The problems of infrastructure decay, facility closure, loss of access, and deterioration of quality described earlier will go unchecked where circumstances limit economic freedom to the freedom to be poor.

Market payment is currently supplanting cost-based reimbursement of capital at a rapid pace. As a result, *reimbursement*, in the strict sense of the term, is becoming less common. Reimbursement implies an extramarket commitment on the part of a buyer to assume responsibility for a provider institution's capital commitments and/or future capital needs. The emerging market relationship between buyers and sellers of hospital services includes no such commitment. Thus, HMOs, PPOs, and other private contractors typically pay hospitals a negotiated, all-inclusive price from which hospitals must extract sufficient profit to meet current capital obligations and save for future capital needs.

Market Payment Proposals for Medicare

Some government entitlement programs and Blue Cross plans—payers that may continue to assume a degree of political or community responsibility for the health of hospitals—also propose to emulate market pricing. They want to do it by replacing capital reimbursement with a standardized capital "payment" that does not recognize individual institutional obligations or needs. This kind of add-on mimics the all-inclusive price arrangement typical of normal private markets, especially when the capital payment is grafted onto a formulaic system for paying operating costs, such as DRGs.

Pressure to eliminate cost-based or need-based reimbursement is particularly strong in the DRG-based Medicare prospective payment system. Continued use of cost-based capital reimbursement in PPS creates a large and inviting cost-control loophole: because operating payments are limited prospectively, hospitals face an incentive to shift as many costs as possible into capital accounts and to substitute capital for labor when labor might be more efficient. Continued cost-based reimbursement of capital also runs counter to the free-market ideology of many political leaders.

When Congress established PPS in 1983, it requested the Department of Health and Human Services to study how best to reimburse capital. When HHS submitted its report (tardily) in March 1986, its conclusions were not unexpected.[12] It recommended that Congress replace cost-based capital reimbursement with a standardized capital payment amount per discharge that would be added to DRG prices. In the meantime, many congressional leaders and interest groups had made similar recommendations, as did the Prospective Payment Commission created by Congress to monitor PPS.[13]

On June 3, 1986, the Health Care Financing Administration published a proposed rule to implement the recommendations of the HHS report. The rule envisioned a standardized capital payment amount per discharge that would be adjusted to account for interhospital differences in geographic location (urban versus rural and by census division), case-mix intensity, indirect medical education costs, and the higher costs of treating a "disproportionate share" of low-income patients.[14] By this time, however, hospitals who would lose funds under prospective capital reimbursement knew who they were and they, along with state and local hospital associations, had had time to organize and lobby against the proposal. Stimulated by this growing opposition, and not wanting HCFA to establish a new capital allowance system without congressional review, Congress quickly asserted its own authority, nullifying the proposed rule and giving itself until October 1, 1987 to establish its own mechanism. But cost savings were still needed to reduce the federal deficit, so Congress substituted an across-the-board percentage reduction in cost-based capital reimbursement: 3.5 percent in fiscal year 1987, 7 percent in fiscal year 1988, and 10 percent in fiscal year 1989.

In May of 1987, HCFA prepared to publish a new Notice of Proposed Rulemaking that set forth a modified version of its previous prospective capital payment proposal. Designed to be implemented in October of 1987, the new proposal responded to earlier criticisms with a number of technical amendments, including a ten-year transition period for plant and fixed equipment. Whether some form of prospective capital payment would be imposed in 1987, either by HCFA or by Congress, remained most uncertain, though. As Chip Kahn, minority staff member to the Senate Finance Committee, told the National Council of Health Facilities Finance Authorities meeting in Philadelphia on May 14, "there is no constituency for efficiency." Although many Democratic leaders in the key House and Senate committees favored or did not oppose prospective capital payment, lobbying from adversely affected hospitals pressed strongly on them. These members were wondering whether prospective principles are worth the fight, according to Kahn, when Congress's first priority—budget savings—could be realized with continued across-the-board cuts that would produce no readily identifiable losers. Indeed, in its December 1987 budget bill, Congress again delayed implementation of prospective capital payment, prohibiting HCFA from implementing its program until fiscal year 1992. Congress instead substituted deeper across-the-board cuts in cost-based reimbursement: 12 percent starting January 1, 1988 and 15 percent in fiscal year 1989.

For the industry as a whole, the long-run impact of across-the-board cuts in cost-based reimbursement may not differ greatly from true prospective payment. Downsizing cost-based capital reimbursement shares fundamental similarities with explicit prospective or market payment of capital: both approaches signal the demise of Medicare's historic commitment to underwrite hospital capital investment, both decrease incentives to invest, and both strenghthen the link between the ability to invest with the ability to make a profit.

In the next section we analyze the likely impact of a shift by Medicare and other payers to market payment using flat rates or standard allowances. We take as our model the recent HCFA designs to standardize Medicare's capital payments.

FLAT-RATE CAPITAL ALLOWANCES

An analysis of flat-rate capital payment[16] and related policies should proceed on two levels. The question of programmatic efficiency—whether or not a particular policy will "work" in a narrow operational sense—should occupy one level of discourse; most of what has been published and said about flat-rate payment adopts the narrow, technical approach appropriate to this question. In addition, behind the programmatic issue lies another, probably more important, question about the evolution of the nation's health care system and how flat-rate payment would affect its development. This question remains largely unspoken and unheeded in the debate over Medicare capital payment policy. The following analysis of flat-rate payment evaluates both its programmatic efficiency and the long-run strategic impact of the policy on health system development.

Practicality

Flat-rate payment, including the standardized payment amount approach developed by HCFA, breaks the connection between capital needs and capital expenditures, on the one hand, and capital reimbursement, on the other. It mimics the way unregulated businesses get paid. Therefore, many proponents believe that flat-rate capital payment of hospitals will promote efficient management, produce a more efficiently structured medical service delivery system, and be simple to design and administer. Ease of administration is an apparent strength of flat-rate payment. Nothing could be simpler than to increase existing reimbursement payments for operating costs by a standardized amount. The bureaucratic and legal mechanisms are in place, and the necessary information is at hand. Simplicity has its side effects, however.

One of these side effects is "mismatch." Hospitals vary widely in the percentage of total expenditures they devote to capital. Proprietary hospitals and hospitals that have recently added beds are well above average in capital expenditures, while large urban public hospitals, teaching hospitals, and hospitals serving large Medicaid populations are below.[17]

Far greater variation separates individual institutions. A recent econometric study by the American Hospital Association included 19 explanatory variables but left more than 70 percent of capital-related cost variation unexplained.[18] A fair and efficient policy ought to recognize much of this variation, both explained and unexplained, yet no formulaic system can hope to do as well as the AHA model. Yet, even an inadequate set of adjustments sacrifice much of the simplicity that is flat-rate payments' most attractive feature, since ease of design and administration deteriorate as the formula becomes complex.

One group of hospitals that will fare especially poorly under flat-rate payment are those that, because of recent renovation or other factors, are obligated to make high annual principal and interest payments on loans. Three options exist to accommodate such hospitals: cost-based coverage of historical obligations, "borrowing forward" from future formulaic payments, or a gradual blending of cost-based and formula-based capital reimbursement.[19] Borrowing forward against future capital reimbursement payments is unrealistic because the future revenue environment, for most hospitals, is too uncertain to attract lenders. Cost-based reimbursement is feasible, but it would be cumbersome to administer because of the regulations and hospital-specific data analysis that would be required for decades into the future. It would also perpetuate the flawed cost-based system. Supporters of flat-rate payment therefore favor blending.

Blending would phase in percentage payment by gradually decreasing the share of total capital reimbursement calculated on a cost basis. If only expenditures for major plant and fixed equipment were allowed to enter the cost-based portion of the blend, then overinvestment due to continued cost-based reimbursement could be controlled.[20] However, if hospital revenues did not rise rapidly, hospital capital obligations would not decrease rapidly as a proportion of total revenues, and many hospitals might become insolvent.[21]

Despite this risk, blending offers a feasible technical fix for the problem of accommodating hospitals that carry large capital repayment obligations. No equivalent fix can compensate for other perverse side effects of flat-rate payment, however. These include other forms of mismatch, such as flat-rate payment's inability to address the needs of institutions that serve the poor, a failing that also violates a second basic criterion of payment system performance—equity.

Equity

As discussed in Chapter 1, financial condition may exclude 50 percent or more of the nation's hospitals from access to private capital markets for major projects. Severe financial distress in most hospitals appears to be caused primarily by the demographics of the neighborhoods they serve, not by poor management or lack of community need. In rural areas and in urban neighborhoods where patients lack sufficient insurance or depend on low-reimbursing Medicaid programs, hospital revenues suffer. In the future, competition and intensified cost control will exacerbate this problem.

If flat-rate payment were set at the current average rate of capital payment in the Medicare program, about 7 percent of operating costs, it would increase reimbursement to distressed hospitals. (Most of these institutions have not been able to invest at a rate that would bring them to the 7 percent national average, even though reimbursement in the past would pay for any capital expenditures a hospital could make. Lack of working capital and pressing operational and community needs consumed available funds, instead.) However, the extra 2 percent or so that financially distressed hospitals would receive under a 7-percent flat-rate payment would not cover the annual operating deficits many of them have.[22] Since their financial future is so threatening, moreover, few if any could enter the debt market on the strength of this small and uncertain additional revenue stream; even substantial extra payments would be unlikely to make them creditworthy.[23] Furthermore, unless some planning mechanism were instituted to focus augmented rates, extra payments would also waste money on those financially distressed hospitals for which no need exists. Not all financially distressed institutions are essential community providers, and not all are well managed.

Efficiency

The short-run efficiency of flat-rate payment is a function of two variables—the investment behavior it induces and its ripple effects on institutional and clinical management.

Much of the support for flat-rate capital payment arises because of the discretion it gives hospital administrators in the selection and financing of capital purchases. Is it correct to assume that managerial discretion will ensure truly efficient hospital behavior? Hospital managers of the future, like those of today, will try to key their future investments to the constraints and incentives imposed by their internal and external operating environments. These environments are far from economically neutral. Frequently, perhaps characteristically, they fail to reward investment according to its productivity in fostering health.

Inside the hospital, the administrator must contend with a fractionated decision structure dominated by physicians who enjoy independent bases of economic and political influence. To maintain the flow of insured patients necessary for the hospital's financial survival, the administrator must work actively to attract and retain physicians, in part by satisfying their often idiosyncratic demands for capital equipment.[24] While the growing supply of physicians and their rapidly progressing incorporation into HMOs, PPOs, and other managed care systems will decrease physician autonomy, hospitals may never be able to ignore the preferences of key fee-for-service physicians. In addition, hospitals will now have to please the care management firms that contract for their business, and up-to-date facilities and a reputation for quality may be as important as price in attracting contracts. In major teaching hospitals, the power of eminent service chiefs (who command multimillion dollar "dowries" when they join an institution) seems likely to persist indefinitely.[25]

The administrator's external environment also will discourage efficient allocation. The need to maintain institutional financial health in an overbedded and highly competitive environment, especially when coupled with the active pursuit of profits in proprietary and aggressive voluntary hospitals, will lead administrators to concentrate investment in the most remunerative services and in the wealthier and better-insured geographic areas. Community-oriented services that cannot be successfully priced or sold, or that serve no marketing purpose, may be ignored entirely.

By lumping capital reimbursement with price-controlled operating cost reimbursement, flat-rate payment makes the hospital's ability to innovate, renovate, and survive entirely dependent on its ability to extract surplus revenues from the pricing system. Flat-rate capital payment will therefore magnify the incentives presented by price control systems such as DRG payment and selective contracting.

Many of these incentives are perverse. In the Medicare DRG system, for example, flat-rate capital payment should strengthen existing incentives toward excess admissions, cost shifting to nonregulated payers, reclassification of patients into more remunerative pricing categories ("DRG creep"), and shifting of assets and costs into nonregulated corporate entities and markets.[26] In addition, because real capital obligations change very little in the short run as occupancy changes, flat-rate payment authorizes extra payments when new capital is needed. This is all to the good in normal businesses, where increased volume signifies a good product and a strong economy. In health care, however, the low marginal cost of additional admissions creates a strong incentive to provide unnecessary care, a practice that subjects patients to unnecessary risks and discomfort, distorts the candor and trust that should characterize the physician-patient relationship, and adds to health care costs. At the same time, responsible hospitals that decrease utilization and costs are penalized. The Reagan administration's proposal for payment by a single, per-hospital amount per discharge intensifies this adverse incentive by overpaying for capital in low-cost DRGs: it rewards hospitals that concentrate on low-cost, rapid-turnover admissions and avoid the sicker patients whose hospital stays are longer.

Strategic Efficiency and Equity: The Longer Run

As long as flat-rate payment of capital remains in effect, the shorter-run problems identified above will continue to hurt rural, poor, and minority areas, promote inefficient investment, and stimulate excess admissions and other managerial inefficiencies. Over time, these processes will help create a national health care infrastructure that is dramatically less equitable and efficient. In addition, the nation will begin to notice other adverse medium- and long-run effects.

One medium-range problem derives from another form of mismatch. Flat-rate payment contains no mechanism (short of grafting on a planned payment component) to provide capital access to hospitals that need to make big-ticket capital expenditures in the decade after flat rates begin. This group includes institutions with pressing renovation needs, such as hospitals constructed during the early Hill-Burton years that are nearing the end of their capital cycle and hospitals located in areas of rapid population growth. Capital-related outlays by these hospitals will need to increase dramatically—to perhaps 15 percent to 20 percent of operating costs or more—during the immediate postinvestment years.[27]

Few, if any, hospitals will be able to cover the difference between these percentages and the 7 percent or less they will receive from flat-rate payment. "Borrowing forward" to the time when flat-rate payments will exceed institutional repayment obligations seems ruled out by the uncertain future reimbursement environment and by the large carrying costs of such borrowing. "Saving up" takes too long and, as we have seen, only very prosperous hospitals seem able to do it. Hospitals owned by large national chains—especially members of for-profit corporations whose shareholders may be willing to take the risks that scare lenders away—may stand a somewhat better chance. Their parent corporations may elect to take years of early losses in the hope of many more years of profits later on. But for-profit hospital management companies have performed poorly in the stock market since the introduction of PPS. They seem to be taking their capital clout outside the hospital sector.

Therefore, if flat-rate payment is to deal with the capital replacement needs of this group of aged hospitals—a group in which financially distressed hospitals are prominent—some special mechanism must be grafted on. HCFA's 1986 proposed rule mentioned the possibility of reducing regular payments to hospitals by 5 percent to 10 percent to create a pool of funds to assist hospitals that were "financially disadvantaged" by a transition to flat-rate payment.[28] Access to the pool would be governed by an "exceptions procedure" based on three quantitative thresholds: a debt-equity ratio greater than 2.00, a ratio of capital expense to flat-rate payment revenue greater than 2.00, and a ratio of annual Medicare payments to Medicare patient expense of less than 1.00.[29] (The last criterion presumably is intended to reward efficient management.) One could debate the specific thresholds proposed by HCFA, but the major problem with formulaic criteria like these is that not all the nation's aged hospitals ought to be replaced and not all are adequately managed, including some (meeting HCFA's third criterion) that keep their costs low enough to make a profit from Medicare. Allowing financial distress alone to trigger extra payment thus defeats a major purpose of both flat-rate payment and planned payment.

It is hard to imagine a formula administered from HCFA's offices in Baltimore that would be capable of distinguishing the deserving from the nondeserving. A justification for replacement depends on complex and incommensurable factors like the relative locations and capacities of neighboring hospitals, commitments to community service and specific populations, quality of care, and consistency with larger local priorities and policies. Any reform of flat-rate payment capable of accommodating most hospitals that face immediate major investment needs must include a planning mechanism if it is to recognize these factors. Community decision making is required to assess community need and programmatic efficiency, lest a blank check be issued to every interested hospital. Such judgments require intimate awareness of community needs and a coordinated local mechanism to negotiate affordable solutions.

In the longer run, most hospitals probably will come to face the same lack of capital access that poor hospitals, and hospitals facing immediate renovation and expansion needs, face now. Increasing competition among hospitals and increasing cost cutting by employers, insurers, and care management corporations can be expected to eliminate easy access to private capital markets for nearly all hospitals. Presidential and congressional attempts to lower the level of flat-rate capital payments will accelerate this process, as will any attempt to accommodate the special needs of certain hospitals, by diverting funds from the regular capital payment stream, as HCFA proposes. It is thus difficult to see any time in the future when flat-rate payment will permit major renovations or expansions to occur without additional subsidization. Ultimately, political pressure will build for new programs to assist construction. The nation's public hospitals already call for a new grant program to finance their rebuilding needs.

Does It Matter?

The United States is, in the aggregate, overbedded. Utilization of existing beds is dropping rapidly. A contraction in capacity seems justified. Why worry that the same pressures that exclude most hospitals from capital markets should cause many hospitals to curtail their services or close their doors? Is this not a solution, rather than a problem? Other hospitals will delay renovation and spend less when they do rebuild, in part to offer lower prices to the PPOs, HMOs, and other price-conscious care managers of the future. Is this not additional evidence that a dose of market discipline has long been needed? Does not flat-rate payment simply allow the market to bring much-needed efficiency to a heretofore undisciplined system?

There obviously is a need for somewhat fewer and more prudently constructed beds and hospitals, but there must be fairer and more efficient ways to satisfy this need. Contraction and delay will occur first and fall most heavily on the areas and institutions which–from a health point of view, in terms of physical deterioration and potential for operating efficiencies, and for equity's sake–deserve more, not less access to capital. By letting profitability determine hospital location, we inherit the same difficulties that analysts and victims of physician location in the United States have long lamented: we have plenty of doctors, they just do not live in the right places. If the process of capacity reduction can be likened to burning a candle, flat-rate payment lights the wrong end.

It also is far from clear that radical capacity contraction is a desirable goal in the emerging competitive era. First, competition requires a certain degree of excess capacity, otherwise patients and purchasers cannot "take their business elsewhere." One or two major closures in many communities would create a very tight market, indeed. After the shakedown, prices will rise again, because entry into the market is highly restricted. Moreover, economic shakedowns affect much more than stock prices and management careers when essential human services are involved. Continuity of care is an important criterion of performance at the institutional and geographic levels as well as at the level of individual patient care.

We also no longer need fear the Roemer effect—the tendency, under historical-cost reimbursement health insurance, for excess capacity to create its own demand. DRGs, global budget rate setting, and capitation—the reimbursement systems of the future—weaken the Roemer effect as recent declines in hospital utilization and occupancy show. Planners and policy makers lambasted excess capacity long and hard for three decades. They did so to a large extent because they lacked the political power to tackle the real problems, which were and are the structure of the health care system and the way we compensate individual and institutional providers. So they attacked what they could and what existing institutions and trade associations had an anticompetitive interest in helping them attack—excess capacity. There seems little point now in continuing to wage this particular "last war," especially when winning would create more problems than leaving well enough alone.

A final reason why radical bed reduction and facility closure are less useful than they seem is that the capital costs of excess capacity are sunk and unrecoverable. The contractors and equipment suppliers have already been paid, and the lenders must be paid regardless of what happens to the plant and equipment. There are rarely alternative uses for hospitals that could attract purchasers willing to pay anything like their replacement costs, and the amount by which the carrying costs of existing debt in excess facilities could be reduced by resale represents a miniscule fraction of a community's annual hospital care bill. The accelerating AIDS epidemic reminds us that there soon may be times when vacant beds will come in handy. By saving some of the "excess" beds it has, the nation might save billions in new construction costs in the longer run, and the cost of keeping open this option is small. The maintenance cost of excess beds probably could be further reduced by "mothballing" certain institutions. Mothballing portions of institutions would help hospitals reduce their active bed complement, preserve the excess, and still lower overhead sufficiently to stay competitive. A planned, local effort will be necessary to implement and finance mothballing, however.

Thus, the problems that flat-rate capital payment will bring *do* matter, and neither the prospect of a stricter market discipline nor the hope of radical reductions in bed capacity makes up for the imposition of these costs. Beneficial competition will proceed in any event, and widespread hospital closures are neither all that desirable nor likely to occur in the right places. To design a workable capital payment policy, we need to move beyond ideological reasoning and consider concretely the capital-related demands that the future health systems will create.

DESIGNING HEALTH CAPITAL POLICY FOR THE REAL FUTURE

There is a natural tendency, when facing long-term uncertainty and the need to design policies, to portray options in ideologic terms. Thus, many assert that health care is a consumer good to be rationed according to personal wealth and income and that the most promising policies are those that imitate classical economic markets. To analysts with this starting point, flat-rate capital payment looks very attractive. As the foregoing analysis shows, however, economic theory founders to a great extent on the rocks of real-world health system structure and behavior. In the past and still today, others start from the assumption that only a centrally planned, publicly managed health care system can be successful. This view seems equally unrealistic.

The recourse to ideology probably arises from several sources. One is laziness: thinking about the future in concrete terms is *hard work*. So is sifting through the past to find its almost-forgotten lessons. So is thinking concretely about institutional design. Ideology is easier, but it is less helpful in the long run.

Selective vision explains another part of the phenomenon of ideological thinking. It is remarkable, in reviewing the health capital predictions of health policy leaders and thinkers over the last 50 years, the extent to which their (mistaken) predictions of the future mimicked their current dreams.

We describe in Chapter 3 how Hill-Burton and other postwar programs created incentives and political structures that destroyed any possibility of achieving the very regionalized hospital system that motivated most, perhaps all, of Hill-Burton's designers. Similarly, the advocates of areawide planning who wrote the AHA's 1969 statement of financial requirements for hospitals and secured its passage took a step that, in retrospect, destroyed all possibility of meaningful community control of hospitals for at least two decades. Larger political and economic forces might have created both these results in any event. The point is that hope and history can blind us to the future. It is easy to organize our understanding of the future in the terms we use to understand the present and past. Blindness is worth fighting against, however, and we have accumulated some history and some policy analytic skills over the years to help us resist. We should use them.

The third attractiveness of ideological thinking is political. Ideology provides a banner under which disparate political armies may assemble on the field of battle. Wishful ideological predictions help motivate and direct the troops. The wide swings that characterized health capital policy in the past reflect the surging advance and retreat of class and party interests. Examples include the shift from private philanthropic support of private voluntary hospitals to governmental support of public hospitals during the New Deal; the sea change after World War II from politically managed intergovernmental subsidies to technically managed transfers of tax funds to private institutions; and the shift from liberal to radically conservative health policies during the first six years of the "Reagan Revolution." One plays King Canute[30] with the long waves of fundamental political change at one's peril—yet many would agree that, like national defense, health care also is "too important to play politics with." Our health care system is mature and well developed, although changing rapidly in response to market forces. It cannot be torn down to start again. Rather, it needs better management, and some sophisticated tinkering—including capital payment and community planning systems realistically designed to work in the real future that awaits them. Since the system is evolving rapidly now and a precise prediction of the future is impossible, we especially need capital and planning policies that can *respond effectively to continuing change.*

Present capital decisions cast a long shadow. Irreversible long-term commitments based on short-term thinking or mistaken forecasts could have tragic opportunity costs. It seems essential that capital policy preserve as much flexibility as possible so it can adapt to future developments. Like the planning systems used by successful private corporations,[31] the nation needs a capital allocation mechanism that forms long-term strategies, can revise them every year, and does not destroy its infrastructure base in the pursuit of short-term administrative or budgetary objectives.

Flat-rate payment provides little flexibility. It removes virtually all control over the details of system evolution from both Congress and local political structures, whether business coalitions, planning agencies, or government. It sets the system's course according to formula and launches it on a radical developmental course. It sends the nation's health system into uncharted waters on automatic pilot.

There is no reason why even ardent supporters of increased competition in health care should feel compelled to flip this switch. Despite the natural affinity between competitive policies and flat-rate payment, flat rates are not necessary to achieve a competitive future. The efficiency of managed care and vertically integrated systems of care – if they are efficient – will assure their ultimate success on the basis of operating cost savings alone. It is not necessary to endure the costs of a technically inefficient and inequitable flat-rate capital payment system to enjoy the benefits of constructive economic competition.

Designing an Alternative

What sort of capital payment system can be designed to fit the real health system future that we face? In the near term, that future of intense competition among providers and packagers of managed care services will transform the capital and institutional structure of the health care system. An alternative capital payment system must come to terms with this competitive, corporate future. It should accept society's current judgment to support or at least tolerate these changes, on the working assumption that greater competition will perform more effectively than past arrangements. A good alternative payment design will provide a base that can adapt to longer-run changes as well. In particular, it should provide some basic, reliable starting point for greater voluntary and governmental control if this turns out to be desirable and politically acceptable.

Acceptance of an at least partially competitive future implies an ameliorative or balance-wheel role for capital payment – compensating from competition's adverse side effects and performing tasks that competition, by design, cannot or should not undertake. A better system would perform this balance-wheel role without ushering in the problems that would accompany widespread flat-rate payment or creating others that are equally destructive, and it would do so while respecting and protecting the integrity of competitive markets where they work. It should not allow its support to preserve institutions that really ought to close, or to promote unfair or inefficient competition through thoughtless subsidization. Rather than building a shelter for obsolete organizational forms, it should construct a greenhouse for essential and innovative organizations and for services that the market itself cannot support.

Accordingly, we propose six objectives or missions that an alternative capital payment system ought to be designed to achieve. They are limited objectives—we cannot expect capital policy to shore up all of competition's soft spots and sagging beams. It cannot do much toward assuring that consumers have sufficient information about care manager performance, for example, although information also is essential if the market is to work. It cannot single-handedly solve the problem of the uninsured or, under a system of exacting experience rating, the uninsurable. But it may be able to accomplish important objectives that relate more directly to capital investment, institutional innovation, and the provision of specific institutional services.

Objective 1: Maintain an accessible and efficient capital infrastructure and preserve society's investment in health capital. Society has an obvious interest in maintaining much of the health capital infrastructure it has purchased. It has a particularly strong interest in preserving institutions that provide essential services to a community, services which would be lost if the institution closed its doors or allowed itself to deteriorate physically and technologically. Often these institutions are called sole community providers, but the problem is not limited to rural or isolated community hospitals, as the term itself and recent Medicare reimbursement policy seem to assume. Hospitals willing and able to serve poor and minority clients in multihospital communities are equally essential and equally under siege. So are many nonhospital institutions. In Boston, for example, large areas of the city have few or no primary care physicians in private or outpatient clinic practice. Since the 1960s, Boston's neighborhood health centers have provided essential, lifesaving care that would not otherwise have been available.[32]

An effective capital payment policy for the future, therefore, ought to continue society's capitalization of these institutions by supporting renovation, replacement, and the acquisition of new technology when internal resources and credit are insufficient. Subsidization of operating costs to keep such institutions open during periods of environmentally imposed insolvency also should be considered, resources permitting. The preservation and maintenance of essential community institutions advance fundamental social goals, including equity of access to health care services and the increased health that access provides; the capacity to respond to AIDS and other epidemics and disasters; and the economic savings that accrue from preventing illness and from detecting it at earlier stages. An additional benefit of preserving essential community providers will be the preservation of the resources that society has invested in these institutions over decades of philanthropy, generous government reimbursement, and support by community-based, formerly tax-exempt Blue Cross plans.[33]

Objective 2: Launch and support essential services that existing markets cannot supply. Markets are hard pressed to provide services at optimal prices, volume, variety, and quality when either producer organizations or consumers have difficulty capturing or recognizing the benefits that services provide. For example, when HMO enrollment turnover is high – it approximated 50 percent in the advanced Twin Cities market in 1986 – HMOs cannot capture the long-run lower costs that effective preventive screening and early treatment eventually provide. Similarly, no producer has an economic interest in providing free services to the indigent, in enrolling or treating patients whose cost of care will exceed the revenues they bring in, or in maintaining quality of care when its deterioration is invisible to its customers.[34] No insurance firm or government entitlement program pays hospitals, nursing homes, and other institutions to cooperate in creating continuity of care and emotional support for patients who move back and forth between various caregivers – for the cancer patient, as an example, who may move between home care, hospice care, and hospital care.

Similarly, hospitals and HMOs can rarely capture the benefits of activities that improve their community more than their enrollees or admittees, yet community services like nutrition, de-leading, epidemiologic research, pest control, and hypertension screening may bring greater payoffs for health than palliative services that are more easily sold.[35] Many of these community-oriented public health services are now provided by government, but experts see advantages in coordinating them through providers of primary care. This is the vision embodied in the term "community-oriented primary care" or COPD. Despite some subsidized successes like the East Boston Neighborhood Health Center, a recent Institute of Medicine report reveals that COPD has not flourished in the current reimbursement environment.[36] It will flourish even less with greater competition.

Education and research may soon become big losers for many hospitals and care management organizations, as well. Yet these functions are vital to the long-range effectiveness and availability of health services. If they can no longer survive on the basis of cross-subsidization from health services reimbursement, direct and carefully planned support will be essential.

We propose, therefore, that a major role for an alternative capital allocation system would be to help support essential services and functions for which market relationships cannot take responsibility. This is an extension of the notion of capital from the usual bricks-and-mortar definition to one that includes all forms of social "infrastructure" that advance health. The identification of which services to support, and where, would be one of the payment system's major activities. Each state's needs will differ, depending on factors such as the existence of free care–bad debt pools, disease patterns, available governmental and private programs, and its sources and amounts of capital funds.

As the definition of capital and infrastructure broadens to include a variety of institutions, services, and processes vital to community health, the question of the acute general hospital's future importance to health infrastructure must be addressed. Progressive businesses and other private sector purchasers of health services, as well as government, rely more and more on care management organizations—rather than independent hospitals and physicians—to manage their health care expenditures. They do so because care managers are better equipped and organized to take responsibility for the continuous and efficient maintenance of an individual's health. If the commercial stratum of the health system is abandoning traditional hospitals as a mechanism to manage care, does it make sense to support their independent recapitalization in the future?

It is by now obvious that the traditional hospital offers an incomplete base on which to maintain either individual health or community health. Unlike an HMO or a public health department, hospitals are organized to sell services and provide curative care in life-threatening illness. The comprehensive health planning movement of the late 1960s made this point strongly. Of course, hospitals have expanded into ambulatory care and other areas of service since the days of CHP. Some have started or established close ties with HMOs. A few take community responsibilities as seriously as finances permit. Nevertheless, it was still accurate in 1985 to say that

> [t]oday, a hospital can meet every legal and accreditation standard without giving any consideration to the community: without knowing the health indices of the community, such as the leading causes of death and disease, or whether the infant mortality rate has bottomed out or is rising . . . Today, most hospitals are as backward with respect to systematic approaches to their community health responsibilities as hospitals were with respect to systematic approaches to controlling quality in 1919. . . .[37]

Despite their limitations, however, hospitals will be an essential component in any future community-oriented health care system. As Bruce Vladeck reminds us,

> [a]s the only care-giving institution in many communities whose doors are open twenty-four hours a day, seven days a week, the hospital takes on a number of additional, residual functions that are vital to community well-being. The paradigm is the emergency room of any large city hospital at

> two o'clock on a Sunday morning when it becomes, in essence, the reception point for every social problem that no other institution can deal with . . . problems of mental health, substance abuse, social displacement, family violence, and criminal justice. Nowhere else are trained professionals and a relatively secure environment available around the clock.[38]

Hospitals serve their communities as "institutions of last resort" in numerous ways, from housing patients unable to gain admittance to nursing homes, to caring (with their many empty beds) for the growing population of AIDS victims, to their long-standing role as providers of free acute care services. As during the era of areawide planning—and since—they often shun this role or play it thoughtlessly and therefore poorly. But unlike doctors, economic prosperity, and investor capital, hospitals sink deep roots in their communities. Most of the nation's HMOs and care management firms lack any roots at all in voluntarism; most are investor-owned. Although they are taking over the management of health care in the United States, these organizations assume no responsibility to care for the indigent, for example. Robert Sigmond,[39] Bruce Vladeck,[40] and others see the embers and occasionally the open flame of a commitment to community health and cooperation in the nation's community hospitals, with their more than 100,000 trustees and their many other volunteers and donors. Any effort to provide community services must include community hospitals and improve them.

Objective 3: Identify and strengthen a cooperative sector within the health services industry. As Rashi Fein wrote in his recent study of national health insurance policy,

> it is useful to have parts of our society and economy that are organized in ways that strengthen our solidarity with others, our charitable instincts, our sense of cooperation. Even as those who would nurture such sectors recognize that America cannot be a Brook Farm or Israeli kibbutz writ large, they would strive to keep health care from turning into just another industry. Those who believe that competition expresses an attitude and value system and does not merely describe a form of economic organization are distressed to see the free market invade one more sanctuary.[41]

Michael Walzer makes a similar point when he divides U.S. society into four domains—business, government, family, and the "cooperative sector"—each with its characteristic mode of action. If coercion is the characteristic activity of government, and commerce of business, cooperation characterizes—or should characterize—the voluntary, community-oriented, nonprofit organizations of society.[42] Historically prominent within the cooperative sectors were hospitals and other provider institutions, although in recent years the hospice movement fit the cooperative model much more faithfully.

Other authors, such as Richard M. Titmus[43] and Kenneth J.

Arrow,[44] have emphasized society's need to preserve means of exchange and interaction other than market relationships, and our persistent tendency to assume that health is "different" from other economic sectors. As Arnold S. Relman argued recently in an exchange with Uwe E. Reinhardt, while a person's relationship with a physician bears resemblances to his or her relationship with a mechanic—in both cases, the person's technical capacity to evaluate the provider's work is limited—the "ethical physician's obligations to his patient go far beyond that."[45]

Sigmond believes we should set higher standards of conduct for community or voluntary hospitals, and use incentives such as tax exemption, access to philanthropy, and capital subsidization to distinguish the cooperative sector from the commercial.[46] In some areas, Medicaid programs, local government, and philanthropy are supporting the creation of HMOs that are willing and able to service the uninsured and uninsurable. A capital payment system appropriate to the competitive future probably should condition much of its support on a commitment to communitywide health and to institutions that cooperate with other community-oriented providers.

Objective 4: Stimulate experimentation and innovation in the organization and delivery of services. Markets are effective stimulators of certain kinds of innovation, but they have been known to retard innovation as well. In the social sector, it requires special effort to promote innovation because insurers and government buyers typically condition reimbursement on adherence to a proven, existing service model. Funds to prime the pump of innovation are, therefore, needed. Capital payment in the future should seek out innovations and ventures that need extramarket support to prove or disprove their worth.

Objective 5: Strengthen and broaden community capacity to plan and act. Community networks and polity represent a form of infrastructure more precious by far than bricks and mortar. Rochester's renowned tradition of community leadership is only partly attributable to its concentrated corporate structure. Rochester has been building its capacity for governance since the community chest era of the 1920s, and has benefited from able leadership over the years. Grants from the Commonwealth Fund in the 1940s established a standing committee structure that may still be seen in the Rochester Area Hospitals' Corporation (see Appendix A). In Boston, a long tradition of enlightened support for community health centers has kept these institutions going during difficult times, preserved community control, and added measurably to the health of the city's residents.[47] The need to act overtakes a community quickly: the capacity to act takes years, probably decades, to build.

Personal and institutional ties must be established and passed on. A shared sense of community must develop before narrower affiliations and interests can be restrained and before the restraint can be justified by results.

A capital payment mechanism that encourages local decision making and keeps local institutions under local control should help preserve and increase community capacities to plan and act. Responsibility breeds capacity.

Objective 6: Preserve and promote effective competitive markets. The importance of compensating for competition's defects without preventing its successes has already been discussed. In addition to avoiding interference in well-functioning competitive markets, a better capital payment system might target its capital funds to preserve the diversity of sellers necessary to foster market competition. The intense competition now erupting in health care is fed to a large degree by the excess hospitals, physicians, and other resources that past policies and community support have produced. A significant continuing amount of excess physical capacity will be required if effective competition is to continue. In some areas, capital support may be necessary to keep this additional capacity on-line.

Capital subsidies can foster competition in another way as well. Currently, hospitals with newer plants are at a competitive disadvantage due to their higher debt retirement obligations. This disadvantage has little or nothing to do with their inherent economic efficiency, and efforts in such hospitals to meet their competitor's prices could hurt quality of care and community service. Thus over the long run, independent community support of capital requirements could help level the "playing field" among competing hospitals while maintaining modern facilities and protecting quality of care.

The Alternative: Planned Payment

The six objectives described above boil down to three basic missions: (1) maintain and improve the health infrastructure of communities, broadly defined; (2) nurture and defend a cooperative or community-oriented stratum alongside the dominant competitive stratum; and (3) support and protect the integrity—and therefore the efficiency—of competitive health care markets where they operate equitably and effectively.

Formula-based capital allowances share with historical-cost reimbursement the characteristic that payments flow from payers directly and automatically to individual institutions, without any intervening reallocation and without passing through any other controlling hands. There are rules to calculate or limit how much money payers send to institutions, but apart from whatever incentives may be consciously built into the rules, the payments are unplanned. Within the rules, payments resemble and certainly are seen by their receiving institutions as entitlements. This is the fundamental drawback of cost-based payments, in addition to the adverse incentives they can create. They entitle institutions, not individuals or communities in need of health care; they invest in a particular mix of inputs, not in the output society really cares about, which is health; and during periods of economic stability, they build the future in the image of the past. When the economic environment is unstable, of course, payment by entitlement pumps capital into institutions that will not survive. When the receiving institutions are oriented toward profit rather than committed to health, automatic payment also offers no mechanism to keep health investment in the health sector, or even in the domestic economy.[48] This wastes the limited resources society can devote to health system renewal and change.

Only one basic alternative to cost-based reimbursement and flat-rate payment of capital exists: planned payment. Broadly speaking, planned payment may be defined as any capital payment mechanism that gives control of funds earmarked for capital purposes to an intervening organization for allocation on some basis other than formula or entitlement. A variety of programs can be designed to meet this definition. It is to a detailed description and evaluation of planned payment options that we now turn.

NOTES

1. Actually, the case could be made that the rich-poor distinction has always been the most important one, at least since 1900. In small town America, which was most of America before 1950, hospitals often shifted ownership to remain solvent. In all their incarnations—public, proprietary, voluntary—they remained primarily community institutions, responsive to community needs and resources. See Peter Buck and Barbara Guttman Rosenkrantz, *Healthy, Wealthy, and Wise* (Cambridge, MA: Harvard University Press, forthcoming).
2. Regina E. Herzlinger and William S. Krasker, "Who Profits from Nonprofits?" *Harvard Business Review* 87 (1987): 93–106.
3. Arnold Relman, "The Future of Medical Practice," *Health Affairs* 2, 2 (1983): 5–19; Arnold S. Relman and Uwe E. Reinhardt, "Debating For-Profit Health Care," *Health Affairs* 5 (1986): 5–31.
4. David Hellman, "Industry Notes," *Hospital Capital Finance* 3, 2 (1986): 7.
5. Donald A. Campbell, "Philanthropy: Shareholders and Capital Formation for Hospitals," *Hospital Capital Finance* 3, 2 (1986): 7–8.
6. Bruce C. Vladeck, "The Dilemma between Competition and Community

Service," *Inquiry* 12 (1985): 115–21; Bruce C. Vladeck, "America's Hospitals," *Health Affairs* 5, 2 (1986): 100–107; Campbell, "Philanthropy."

7. Richard L. Johnson, "The Myth of Dominance by National Health Care Corporations," *Frontiers of Health Services Management* 3 (May 1987): 3–22.
8. Robert E. Patricelli, "Musings of a Blind Man—Reflections on the Health Care Industry," *Health Affairs* 5 (Spring 1987): 128–34.
9. Robert Levin, "A Corporate Perspective on Long-Term Care," *Business and Health* 3 (April 1986): 28.
10. Care management systems will market themselves in part on the basis of the reputation, ambience, and accessibility of the hospitals with whom they contract. Moreover, they will want to establish long-term working relationships with hospitals; as hospital capacity contracts, they will find it more difficult to terminate the relationships they have. The cost of constructing new hospital facilities will be prohibitive for most care managers, especially as serious price competition begins in the industry. In the long run, surviving hospitals may gain considerable influence and become full partners in the care management business.
11. Blue Cross, the insurance system created by hospitals to maintain their solvency during the depression, is moving into managed care in many regions as well as nationally, however. Now that Congress has rescinded the Blue Cross federal tax exemption, this offspring of the hospitals' may end up consuming its parent institutions.
12. Office of the Assistant Secretary for Planning and Evaluation, Department of Health and Human Services, *Hospital Capital Expenses: A Medicare Payment Strategy for the Future* (Washington, DC: Office of the Assistant Secretary, 1986).
13. Prospective Payment Assessment Commission, *1987 Adjustments to the Medicare Prospective Payment System*, Report to the Congress (Washington, DC: The Commission, November 1986).
14. *Federal Register* 51 (June 3, 1986) 19,970–20,009, 20,010.
15. Joseph Bower, *Managing the Resource Allocation Process* (Cambridge, MA: Business School, Harvard University, 1972).
16. To avoid semantic clumsiness, we use the term "flat-rate payment" to refer to all variations on the formulaic capital allowance theme. Some proposals call for true "percentage payment," that is, calculating a capital allowance as a fixed percentage of DRG prices or of operating revenues measured in some other way. The HHS proposal is for a fixed payment amount per discharge, which means that capital reimbursement as a percentage of total reimbursement will be higher for low-cost cases and lower for high-cost cases.
17. Gerard Anderson and Paul B. Ginsburg, "Prospective Capital Payments to Hospitals," *Health Affairs* 2 (Fall 1983): 52–63.
18. American Hospital Association, "Capital-Related Cost Variation across Hospitals" (Chicago: American Hospital Association, 1984).
19. Gerard Anderson and Paul B. Ginsburg, "Medicare Payment and Hospital Capital: Future Policy Options," *Health Affairs* 3 (Fall 1984): 35–48.
20. The long construction and repayment periods typical of major projects may help prevent a feeding frenzy because the blending period will attenuate and expire before a significant portion of such major expenditures can be recouped through cost-based payment. (Nevertheless, tax-exempt borrowing jumped dramatically in the year after Congress announced its intention

to fold capital payment into the DRG system. Anxiety that Congress would eliminate tax-exempt financing for hospitals also stimulated the jump.) Alternatively, only repayment and interest obligations incurred prior to the blending period could be allowed, but that would penalize hospitals with low historical obligations.

21. Leonard F. Krystynak, "Prospective Payment for Capital: The Financial Nature of Capital Allowances," *Healthcare Financial Management* (October 1983): 60–76; Leonard F. Krystynak, *Prospective Payment for Capital: The Financial Nature of Capital Allowances* (Oak Brook, IL: Healthcare Financial Management Association, 1983).
22. Nancy M. Kane, "New York City Hospitals: Relationships among Hospital Financial Status, Claimed Capital Need, Likely Capital Access, and Community Characteristics," Health Capital Project Working Paper #6 (Boston: School of Public Health, Harvard University, 1984).
23. Even if very sizable increases in payment rates were channeled to financially distressed hospitals, these hospitals probably would not save the extra funds for major capital investment. In New York City, for example, where effective revenue controls have been in place since the middle 1970s, hospitals as a group have not responded by lowering operating expenditures sufficiently to maintain infrastructure. Approximately 75 percent of New York City's voluntary hospitals do not meet the minimum bond-rating standards required to issue long-term debt, even though public hospitals assume the burden of caring for many of the city's poor. Moreover, these hospitals have invested relatively little in plant and equipment in recent years, and as a result they occupy facilities that are aged and presumably inefficient. See Kane, "New York City Hospitals"; Charles Brecher and Susan Nesbitt, *The Financial Condition of New York City Voluntary Hospitals* (New York: Commonwealth Fund, 1984); and D. McCarthy, "Capital Offense: New York's Health Care in the Crunch," *Health/PAC Bulletin* 14 (1984): 5–14. Similar behavior was observed in voluntary hospitals before the passage of Medicare and Medicaid. See Eleanor D. Kinney and Bonnie Lefcowitz, "Capital Cost Reimbursement to Community Hospitals under Federal Health Insurance Programs," *Journal of Health Politics, Policy and Law* 7 (1982): 648–66.
24. David W. Young and Richard B. Saltman, *The Hospital Power Equilibrium: Physician Behavior and Cost Control* (Baltimore: Johns Hopkins University Press, 1985).
25. Ibid.
26. Henry J. Aaron, "Prospective Payment: The Next Big Policy Disappointment?" *Health Affairs* 4 (Fall 1984): 102–7; R.S. Stern and A.M. Epstein, "Institutional Response to Prospective Payment Based on Diagnosis-Related Groups," *The New England Journal of Medicine* 312 (1985): 621–27.
27. Anderson and Ginsburg, "Medicare Payment and Hospital Capital."
28. *Federal Register* 51 (June 3, 1986): 19,981.
29. The text of the proposed rule calls for a "negative" ratio. This is not mathematically possible in the circumstances: presumably HCFA meant a ratio less than 1.00.
30. For those who may be unfamiliar with the legend, King Canute—thinking himself an absolute monarch—commanded his throne to be placed at the ocean's edge at low tide and then commanded the tide to stay out.
31. Bower, *Managing the Resource Allocation Process*.

32. Bruce Vladeck, "Variations Data and the Regulatory Rationale," *Health Affairs* 3 (1984): 102–9; Vladeck, "The Dilemma."
33. David W. Young, "Ownership Conversions in Health Care Organizations: Who Should Benefit?" *Journal of Health Politics, Policy and Law* 10 (1986): 765–74.
34. The fact that direct purchasers of health services, the insurers and governmental payers, are not the direct beneficiaries of services compounds the problem of market failure with respect to quality of care. This characteristic of medical care markets is frequently cited to explain the "moral hazard" that encourages patients to use more services than they need because they do not bear the direct cost. The converse is equally true, however: major payers are encouraged in a competitive environment to cut insurance coverage, payment, and eligibility excessively because neither they, nor the organizations and professionals they bargain with, lose the direct benefits.
35. For a challenging review of the relative benefits of investing in curative versus preventive services, see Louise B. Russell, *Is Prevention Better than Cure?* (Washington, DC: Brookings Institution, 1986).
36. Institute of Medicine, *Community Oriented Primary Care: A Practical Assessment* (Washington, DC: National Academy Press, 1984).
37. Robert M. Sigmond, "Re-Examining the Role of the Community Hospital in a Competitive Environment," The Michael M. Davis Lecture, Center for Health Administration Studies, University of Chicago, 1985, p. 11.
38. Vladeck, "America's Hospitals."
39. Sigmond, "Re-Examining the Role."
40. Vladeck, "Variations Data"; Vladeck, "The Dilemma."
41. Rashi Fein, *Medical Care, Medical Costs: The Search for a Health Insurance Policy* (Cambridge, MA: Harvard University Press, 1986), p. 192.
42. Michael Walzer, "Toward a Theory of Social Assignments." In Winthrop Knowlton and Richard Zeckhauser, eds., *American Society: Public and Private Responsibilities* (Cambridge, MA: Ballinger, 1986), pp. 79–96.
43. Richard M. Titmus, *The Gift Relationship* (New York: Vintage Books, 1971).
44. Kenneth J. Arrow, "Gifts and Exchanges." In Marshall Cohen, et al., eds., *Medicine and Moral Philosophy* (Princeton: Princeton University Press, 1981), pp. 139–58.
45. Arnold S. Relman and Uwe E. Reinhardt, "Debating For-Profit Health Care," *Health Affairs* 5, 2 (1986): 26.
46. Sigmond, "Re-Examining the Role."
47. See, for example, Dale Young, *A Promise Kept: Boston's Neighborhood Health Centers* (Boston: Trustees of Health and Hospitals, City of Boston, 1982).
48. It may be that the percentage of gross national product devoted to hospital and health care is too high and that shifting resources out of health care would be a good idea. Moving out paid-for capital resources that lack resale value is not an efficient way to accomplish this shift, however.

3.

Planned Payment for Capital and the Community Health Infrastructure Bank

PLANNED PAYMENT FOR CAPITAL

It is important at the outset to distinguish *planned payment,* which is an arrangement to allocate real dollars, from two other activities that history and conventional wisdom closely associate with it—*health planning* and *capital expenditure regulation* (also commonly called certificate of need). Planned payment obviously requires some form of health planning if it is to advance health, but committees can meet and plans be written without planned payment. In fact, planning usually has proceeded in the United States and other Western countries without much control over capital or operating funds. This probably explains its lack of effect.[1]

Unlike planning, capital expenditure regulation does control resources; but, unlike planned payment, it does not allocate capital directly. Instead, it attempts to control the ability of institutions to use their own funds and credit. This is an absolutely crucial difference, with several far-reaching practical ramifications that this chapter will try to clarify. For example, whereas CoN is regulatory and juridical, evolving in some states into a legalistic thicket of remarkable density and profit to lawyers, planned payment is distributive and can operate more on the basis of programmatic innovation and negotiation, selecting projects by comparison rather than according to preset standards. Whereas CoN must regulate all similarly situated institutions equally, planned payment can concentrate on a subset of beneficiaries and coexist more easily with open competition in the rest of the system. These are only two of the important differences.[2]

Despite the necessity to distinguish clearly among planning, planned payment, and regulation, history weaves them together in our experience and imagination. The failures of health planning and regulation consequently cast a deep shadow over new proposals for planned payment of capital. The shortcomings of flat-rate payment detailed in Chapter 2 support planned payment by default, but many health policy experts and leaders would be surprised that a positive case can be made. History teaches that "planning doesn't work." If capital regulation was bad, planned payment will be worse, the reasoning goes.

In fact, the lessons of planned payment's history are not so simple, nor are they so negative. A more sophisticated understanding of history helps distinguish between failures of design and more fundamental failures of concept. If stone arches fall because arches are impossible to build, we should not try to build them. But if they fall because the shape is wrong, or the stones are not set quite right, or the ground is unsteady, we can work at building arches and eventually build cathedrals. A careful look at history helps us distinguish among the different shapes of planning, and it teaches many other lessons useful to the design and evaluation of potential planned payment arrangements.

The next section summarizes this history and its lessons. Following this summary, we extract the basic generic characteristics of a planned payment model that history suggests would be most likely to succeed. We conclude by contrasting this generic model with certificate-of-need regulation of capital expenditures. We show how most of the valid criticisms of CoN are attributable to features of its structure that a well-crafted planned payment system would eliminate. This sets the stage for Chapter 4, in which we propose a specific planned payment institution, one that can coexist with competition and can accomplish the mission described at the end of Chapter 2.

LESSONS FROM THE PAST

Planned health capital payment has been attempted on two occasions in the United States. Hill-Burton represents the first attempt; the second was voluntary areawide planning during planning's brief "golden age." The history of Hill-Burton and areawide planning cannot prove that some new form of planned payment would work in the 1990s, or specify a mission for such a program. History does remind us, however, that planned payment can successfully be embodied in programs. The records of these programs contain lessons about planned payment that designers of new models can use.

Enacted in 1946, Hill-Burton was a program that allocated federal tax dollars to health facility construction in the form of grants awarded on the basis of state-level construction plans. Although very effective at achieving its objectives during its early years—I.S. Falk was later to call it nearly flawless[3]—the program came under increasing fire from a variety of critics and faded away in fairly widespread disrepute in the early 1970s. Areawide planning was a nongovernmental community activity. In cities like Rochester, where it took control of pools of capital funds, areawide planning allocated corporate contributions through needs assessment, performance evaluation, and negotiation. Today, areawide planning is more forgotten than disdained.

The demise of Hill-Burton and areawide planning can be traced in part to the way they were designed and in part to unforeseen changes in their political and economic environments. During the relatively brief periods when they matched their environments, both programs succeeded dramatically and were seen to be successful by contemporary observers. Indeed, the greatest design defect of the Hill-Burton program undoubtedly was its inability to respond creatively to changes in the health policy environment. It was a program optimized to solve a single problem—the lack of adequate hospitals in rural areas. That problem disappeared, largely due to Hill-Burton's own success. When Congress tried to apply the original design, without significant modification, to new problems—hospital construction in urban areas, construction of community health centers—and to do so in an overbedded, well-insured health care economy, the old design failed.

Details Matter

The events leading up to Hill-Burton's enactment emphasize how many choices there are in the design of a planned payment program and how important it is to think clearly about how a particular design will function in alternative economic and political environments. Hill-Burton was far more carefully planned than many programs, yet a combination of historical baggage, idiosyncratic postwar politics, economic interest, institutional rivalry, and personal ambition introduced fatal rigidities into Hill-Burton's structure. No doubt, idiosyncratic factors would influence the enactment of any future planned payment program, whether developed by a state legislature or by Congress. But future designers can use the Hill-Burton and areawide planning experience to see more clearly the implications of the choices they are asked to make.

To appreciate the historical baggage that Hill-Burton's initiators carried to Congress in 1946, one must look back 14 years earlier to the New Deal hospital and health care financing programs begun during the depths of the Great Depression. The Roosevelt administration allocated considerable resources to health care during the 1930s, but voluntary hospitals, especially leading hospitals in larger urban areas, saw little federal money. Working through the Work Projects Administration, the Public Works Administration, and other economic recovery agencies, Roosevelt gave large amounts of money to build, expand, or renovate public hospitals owned primarily by city and county government. These same agencies gave additional grants to local health departments, which allocated the funds to sewer and water supply construction, to traditional public health programs such as milk inspection, and–in some localities–to support for the hospitalization costs of indigent patients. The percentage of gross national product spent on medical care increased from 3.6 to 4.1 between 1929 and 1935, as government subsidization made up for declines in private spending.[4] Most of these funds passed directly from federal to local hands, and state governments played a much smaller role than they would have liked. Party politics and ethnic majorities often controlled how the funds were spent. The more patrician, Republican, white Protestant boards that governed many voluntary hospitals could not control these newly empowered political forces and had long disdained them.

A second important item of historical baggage was more intellectual than institutional or political. Medical reformers had long hoped to transform both the practice and the financing of medicine, which they viewed as lagging far behind the frontier of scientific medicine. The 1932 report of the Committee on the Costs of Medical Care encapsulates this view. The majority of the committee sought to improve the quality and lessen the commercialism of medical practice, hasten the dissemination of scientific medical advances, extend the benefits of public health services and medical care to the entire population regardless of economic circumstance, and improve medicine's physical infractructure. They sought to achieve these goals through what Daniel M. Fox calls "hierarchical regionalism," a combination of: (1) clinical leadership and management radiating downward from academic specialist physicians; and (2) a congruent, regional, physical and operational structure for institutions based on geography, patterns of residence, and responsibility for the health of defined populations.[5] In addition to calling for group practice of medicine and the prepayment of medical and hospital care, the majority statement in the committee's controversial final report recommended, as Fox summarizes it, the conversion of

> suitable hospitals into comprehensive health centers, each one serving a geographic area. These centers would be, in the words of the report, the keystone of satisfactory medical service. Each center would consist of a general hospital with inpatient, outpatient, and public health activities . . . [and provide a hub for] branches and medical stations in its region.[6]

The publication of the committee's report mobilized traditional fee-for-service medicine into strong opposition to prepayment. This opposition prevented the enactment of any significant form of governmental health insurance until Medicare in 1965. But the goal of hierarchical regionalism lived on in the minds of the leaders who devised Hill-Burton, as it lives today in the minds of many academic physicians and policy makers.

By the late 1930s, leaders of voluntary hospitals anticipated federal legislation that would subsidize voluntary hospital construction. A bill to construct hospitals, subsidize maternal and child health services, and support children and adults with disabilities was defeated in 1940 because it would have provided grants to states to establish compulsory health insurance programs. So leaders of the U.S. Public Health Service, the hospital associations, and others desirous of governmental financial support changed their strategy. They decided to separate the highly charged issue of how to pay for services from the questions of better physical planning and increased federal support for health activities. They decided, in Fox's words, "to mobilize the [growing] enthusiasm of the public and its elected representatives for medical science on behalf of policies to increase the supply of medical services—of hospitals, of bio-medical research and, eventually, of doctors."[7]

But while they discarded their hopes of reorganizing physician practice and rationalizing payment for medical services, they retained the notion of hierarchical regionalism in planning the expansion of physical facilities. They failed to recognize the contradiction between a regionalized structure for capital and a competitive market structure for both medical practice and medical insurance. In effect, they kept their old image of their goal but set about creating economic incentives that were sure to destroy any possibility that the goal would be realized.[8]

By 1943, the American Hospital Association began to organize broad support for a program to subsidize postwar voluntary hospital construction. Replacement of New Deal and wartime hospital construction legislation was widely anticipated to be part of an effort to reduce unemployment among returning servicemen and to forestall a return of the prewar depression. The AHA created a Postwar Planning Committee under its lobbying arm to make sure that voluntary hospitals were not again excluded from eligibility. In addition, a year later, the AHA organized a Commission on Hospital Care with support from the W.K. Kellogg Foundation and the March of Dimes to document the need for hospital construction and to build support for a federal program. Both of the AHA groups soon joined forces with the U.S. Public Health Service.

Roosevelt had not given the PHS control of the New Deal and wartime hospital construction subsidies (more historical baggage), but its leader, Surgeon General Thomas Parran, hoped to administer any postwar program. Parran must have seen a supportive constituency in the AHA and the broad coalition of interest groups that the AHA was building. This was a new coalition, one that would support his bid to control postwar construction grants. He must have seen in hierarchical regionalism a seemingly nonpartisan ideology to justify PHS control. The PHS could get away with a remarkable degree of independent coalition building and reform mongering because the president, his staff, and the more heavyweight federal agencies remained preoccupied with the war.[9] However, Parran could not introduce legislation himself without executive office clearance, and the legislation he contemplated ran counter to both presidential philosophy and political interest. (Its eventual godfather in Congress, Robert Taft, was preparing to challenge the Democrats for the presidency). Clearance was an impossibility. The AHA gave Parran a way to introduce the bill.

Bureaucratic politics and perhaps personal ambition thus linked up with historical forces and the economic interests of voluntary hospitals to define the structure–and ultimately the effectiveness–of the Hill-Burton Program. At the proper moment, Parran presented draft legislation to the AHA's Postwar Planning Committee and gained the committee's enthusiastic support.[10] But Parran also needed data and technical expertise[11] to justify a need for voluntary hospital construction and to convince Congress that his agency could administer the construction program. He also had "a couple hundred thousand dollars of postwar planning money."[12] The AHA's Commission on Hospital Care, in turn, needed additional financial and technical assistance to field and analyze a questionnaire. In return for assurances that he could present the data to Congress as his own, Parran gave the commission a staff of 20 to code data and the half-time services of a PHS statistician.

The PHS also enjoyed a history of close working relationships with state governments as a result of the public health programs it had administered. Building on these relationships, and on the intense desire of the states to regain control over federal grant funds,[13] the PHS and the AHA Commission on Hospital Care gave grants and loaned personnel to states to survey existing hospital facilities. With additional support from the Kellogg Foundation, the commission undertook a demonstration project in Michigan that developed facility survey and planning methods which other states later adopted.

George Bugbee, the recently appointed AHA executive secretary, registered as a lobbyist in early 1946 and asked an acquaintance from his days as a hospital administrator in Cleveland, Senator Phillip Burton, to introduce the bill.[14] Parran "formally regretted [in testimony before Congress] that he could not endorse the bill because there was no official policy yet on how it related to the President's program, and then accepted suggestions by the bill's supporters for changes in the way the PHS would administer it."[15]

Congressional politics then further modified the program's design. Senator and Republican presidential hopeful Robert A. Taft, Burton's senior senatorial partner from Ohio, needed a "health bill" and undertook to shepherd the legislation through Congress. Taft personally rewrote substantial portions to benefit the poorer, rural, southern, and middle western states whose senators and representatives controlled Congress.[16] He asked I.S. Falk to invent a formula that would accomplish this objective and prevent any subsequent political interference with the division of grants among the states.[17]

Under Taft's leadership, Congress passed the Hospital Survey and Construction Act of 1946—the Hill-Burton program—while the AHA commission was still in the midst of its work. Delighted after so many years of bitter controversy to consider a bill supported by everyone from organized medicine to the veterans of the Committee on the Costs of Medical Care,[18] Congress appropriated $3 million for state surveys and long-range facility plan development and $375 million dollars for five years of health facility construction grants.

The Necessity of Politics

Known in the Senate as "Mr. Republican," Taft's principal objective in rewriting the Hill-Burton legislation, apart from securing passage, was to depoliticize the allocation of federal funds. In a sense, his allocation formula did this, although it would be more correct to say that the formula helped freeze the congressional balance of power as of 1946 and imposed a more Republican style of politics on the allocation process. That Congress did not change the formula for many years thereafter may be due as much to the seniority of Senator Lister Hill of Alabama, who defended the formula in the interest of his relatively impoverished rural state, as to Taft's foresight. Nevertheless, later studies indicated that the combination of Taft's formula and Hill's persistence did succeed in nearly equalizing per capita hospital beds across states.[19]

This accomplishment demonstrates the potential power of planned payment to redirect resources, at least when the top-down, strategic decisions about major flows of funds do not depend on bottom-up requests from potential beneficiaries. When the volume and "quality" of applicants for funds determine how funds are allocated, it is likely that existing patterns of wealth and political power will reproduce themselves. When decisions about the relative flows of funds to classes of beneficiaries are made independently, these decisions can create new holders of wealth and power.[20] The moral for future planned payment designs with a redistributive purpose may be to create two independent levels of allocational decision making: a top-down level that makes strategic decisions about areas of support, and a bottom-up level that selects institutional beneficiaries within each distributional category. Decision makers at the two levels should owe accountability to different configurations of interests. Later on, in Chapter 5, we discuss the pattern of politics that results from such an arrangement and call it "managed pluralism."

Taft introduced other amendments to depoliticize the bill that were less successful in the long run. The bill required each state to allocate funds strictly on the basis of a written annual construction plan, broken down by hospital market regions called health service areas. Construction allocations were to be planned on the basis of relative need—usually, actual beds per capita compared to some standard of needed beds per capita. The bill established numerical bed-need maximums—which most states soon adopted as standards of need rather than limits on need—and broke these standards down into regionalism's classical categories of base, intermediate, and rural areas. Although Hill-Burton gave states considerable latitude in the specification of regions and the creation of the plans, it required every plan, every allocation made under the plan, and every change in an allocation to be approved by the surgeon general. It gave the surgeon general authority to lay down rules to govern the order in which applications from institutions were to be funded under each state's plan, with poorer rural areas getting first priority. Finally, it gave the federal government authority to promulgate detailed construction and equipment standards which each application had to meet before it could receive approval.

This rigid, technical system ensured that rural areas without adequate hospital facilities were among the first recipients of program funds. It worked fairly well in many rural areas that lacked hospitals when, for example, only one group or location applied for funds. When more than one group applied, each proposing a tiny facility and none able to garner support from competing communities, problems arose. Sometimes the state Hill-Burton agency was able to use its control of funds to force communities to negotiate and start working together.[21] On other occasions the agency could select what it considered to be the best application, since priority of funding depended on the ratio of existing plus anticipated beds to needed beds per capita; competing applicants would then fall back in the queue. But the detailed rules defining need and position in the queue limited agencies' ability to bargain, as did a statutory prohibition against interfering in the ongoing operation of hospitals—and what hospitals *do* is always more important to community health than how they are built.[22] The overly generous bed-need standard, combined with the huge appropriations Congress poured into the states each year, further limited agencies' ability to say no: since the agencies were spending "federal money," they were under great pressure to spend each year's allotment fully. They could not credibly threaten to return money to extract reasonable concessions from an applicant. Although amendments to the law beginning in 1954 appropriated funds for additional beneficiary groups, such as nursing homes, educational facilities, and health centers, state agencies never received much discretion to impose discipline by moving significant amounts of funding out of the hospital pool. In the end, hospitals knew the rules, and they simply got in line.

Hill-Burton's rule-laden and formula-bound approach proved even less effective as the delivery system changed, as the completion of construction in rural areas brought urban and suburban hospitals to the head of the queue, and as Congress amended the program to permit more funding for renovation and replacement in addition to new construction. As an expanding economy and widespread health insurance and entitlement allowed hospitals to increase indebtedness (and therefore to finance capital projects without Hill-Burton's aid), overinvestment both threatened the stability of the hospital industry and helped fuel rapidly rising health care costs. Hill-Burton's overly generous bed-need maximum encouraged rather than discouraged overbedding.

The numerical need formulas that served fairly well as a means to locate new construction also lacked relevance to the problem of deciding among renovation projects. Renovation allocations require complex comparisons among alternative institutions and alternative investment plans. Such comparisons are difficult to reduce to a formula because multiple, interactive objectives are at stake and one hospital's actions can strongly affect the desirability of renovation at other institutions. Besides, the agency was required to consider all applications on a first-come, first-served basis, so opportunities to compare investment options were rare. Moreover, by this time Hill-Burton expenditures accounted for less than 10 percent of total construction financing, so agencies lacked the influence to force negotiated solutions.

Hill-Burton could have invested its funds more effectively by delegating decision making to a community planning agency. But, as Anne R. Somers remarked in her perceptive 1969 book, *Hospital Regulation: The Dilemma of Public Policy,*[23] Hill-Burton contained no mechanism to reconcile areawide planning with its own "apolitical," rule-based capital allocation activities. Hill-Burton did contribute funds to voluntary areawide planning organizations on a research and demonstration basis starting in 1962. In 1964, Congress appropriated and earmarked funds for grants to areawide health facilities planning agencies. In some cases, leaders of these organizations also sat on Hill-Burton advisory boards and added Hill-Burton officials to their own boards.[24] However, as Symond R. Gottlieb described the situation, Hill-Burton grants to areawide planning agencies "were administered directly from Washington, and the state agencies were not involved in the process. . . . No attempt was made to tie together the state and local planning or decision-making activities, and it seldom evolved into any structured relationship."[25]

Hill-Burton's mounting difficulties stand in marked contrast to the success of areawide voluntary planning when it controlled the lion's share of capital available to health care institutions. In Rochester, it will be recalled, community control of a hospital fund drive resulted in the closure of two low quality hospitals, their replacement with new facilities under new management, new investment in nonhospital, intermediate care facilities to meet a community need for long-term care, and the strict limitation of acute hospital beds to 3.4 per 1,000 population. Leadership by competent, powerful, and widely respected corporate executives and planning agency staff made this success possible. Equally important was the community's control of a large, but intentionally *limited*, pool of funds, and its ability to shift funds to alternative uses on the basis of need and in response to political and economic opportunities. Moreover, the Rochester community leadership controlled a large enough proportion of the total funds available for construction that it could prevent construction as well as promote it. In communities where areawide planning agencies did not control this sort of pool, their influence appears to have been much less.

Planning for multiple independent organizations raises complex political and substantive issues. It works best when it creates and uses opportunities for collective deliberation and active negotiation. Without areawide planning processes to help them, Hill-Burton agencies found it impossible to promote responsible investment when they ran out of rural areas without hospitals and confronted hospital markets shared by several competitors. By overreacting to the "dirty," partisan politics of New Deal subsidy programs, the framers of Hill-Burton created an ecosystem too abstractly pure to support a diversity of life. This history suggests that new planned payment designs should build political conflict into the allocation process; they should use it to good advantage rather than try—inevitably without success—to exclude politics. They should seek to make the governance of the planned payment organization accountable to the community's true needs and interests, and then minimize the extent to which they constrain this governance with rules, formulas, and legalistic due process requirements.

In addition to creating a limited pool of funds, planned payment can further promote community governance by allowing funds to go unspent indefinitely. A willingness to hold funds until good proposals have been developed will encourage the development of good proposals. A planned payment organization could counter the inevitable pressure to spend available funds by building into its mandate the subsidization of several competing beneficiary groups and by giving itself the authority to shift funds among groups.

Hill-Burton-style prohibitions against involvement in institutional management also seem counterproductive, especially for a planned payment system that attempts to support a "cooperative sector." As Chapters 1 and 2 make clear, the incentives produced by capital payment mechanisms and the operating cost implications of capital investment are both more important than the value of the investment, itself. Future planned payment arrangements should build in mechanisms to encourage desired managerial behavior and enforce behavioral promises made when capital funds are committed. Hill-Burton, for example, was eventually much criticized because it failed to enforce free care commitments it had required hospitals to make when they accepted funds.

The creation of a planned payment governance arrangement that commands respect and truly serves the community interest requires care. Past attempts met with only brief success. Voluntary areawide planning groups also attracted criticism for their dominance by corporate and social elites and close connections with hospital boards. The comprehensive health planning agencies that succeeded them, and their successors, the health systems agencies, demonstrate the futility of overreacting in the other direction. They attempted to substitute "mirror representation" and opportunities for participation for real accountability to organized interests, be they providers, neighborhoods, governments, labor, or business.[26] We analyze the governance problem in more detail in Chapter 5.

The Danger of a Single-Sector Program

Many of the difficulties Hill-Burton encountered arose from an inability to change its rules as well as from the fact that so many rules were used. This stalemate in Congress, in the federal executive branch, and in state government arose to a great extent from another aspect of Hill-Burton's design, its careful targeting of benefits primarily to a single interest group—nonprofit general hospitals.

Through its intimate involvement in the drafting and mark-up sessions, the AHA was able to craft a bill that made voluntary hospitals almost the sole beneficiary, while simultaneously giving political control of the program to the hospital industry. For example, the bill explicitly prohibited any federal officer from exercising "any supervision or control over the administration, personnel, maintenance, or operation of any hospital."[27] Just to be sure that the surgeon general did not by regulation or administrative action interfere with the interests of hospitals, the bill created a private Federal Hospital Council dominated by hospital representatives with power to approve all regulations and to settle institutional and state agency appeals of key administrative actions.[28] Thus, although Hill-Burton is remembered by many as a federal program that gave great autonomy to the states, perhaps Congress granted the real autonomy to the hospitals themselves and to the elite community constituencies that supported them. The rules imposed on state implementing agencies protected the hospital industry's subsidy from political "interference," while a provision that limited federal participation in the financing of any facility to 33 percent[29] made it impossible for a hospital to receive funds without its own philanthropic or governmental financial support. This protected the existing institutions. As discussed, however, there were no provisions for democratic, *areawide* community control.

The Hill-Burton act actually authorized funds for several kinds of facilities in addition to general hospitals—hospitals serving tuberculosis, mental, and chronic-disease patients and public health centers. But when the regulations were published,[30] states were required to give priority to chronic-disease facilities that would be operated as subunits of general hospitals, to locate tuberculosis and mental hospitals close to general hospitals, and to allocate funds among the various institutional groups in proportion to need. Because need tended to be calculated as the difference between existing facility capacity and the federally promulgated "maximum requirements," general hospitals were further advantaged—the maximum requirements were very generous for general hospitals but less so for other facilities. The statewide "requirement" for general hospitals was 4.5 beds per 1,000 persons. Its origin shows the extent to which hospital interests shaped the development of the legislation:

> In executive session, Senator Robert Taft expressed concern to Bugbee and [PHS representative Vance Hoge] that the Hill-Burton Program might fund too many beds. According to Bugbee, he and [Hoge] went back to the Public Health Service office and, after reviewing data, chose the 4.5 figure, fairly certain that the [level] could never be reached. . . .[31]

Proprietary hospitals were made ineligible for Hill-Burton funds and, although the 1947 regulations required states to give priority to the construction of new beds, they encouraged replacement in areas supplied by beds deemed to pose a "hazard." Often, such older facilities in rural areas were proprietary hospitals owned by individual physicians.[32]

The act therefore encouraged new or expanding voluntary facilities to put proprietaries out of business—another long-time objective of the voluntary hospitals. The detailed construction and equipment standards promulgated by the federal government—standards ratcheted up each year by subcommittees of the Federal Hospital Board dominated by architects and equipment manufacturers[33]—accelerated this process. In addition, health service areas, the basic geographic units within which bed need was calculated, were by law and regulation centered around existing large hospitals, which tended to bias planning against upstart facilities at the interstices of planning regions.[34]

Many of these cost- and quality-increasing and anticompetitive effects were seen as genuine reforms, which in part they were, especially in rural areas. Postwar physical facilities and clinical practice cried out for improvement. In the words of the Commission on Hospital Care, "We frequently refer to our splendid system of hospitals, whereas in reality there is none. . . . In most states, anyone can establish the most meagre facility for the bed care of the sick and call it a hospital."[35] But the tight exclusive pairing of voluntary hospital interests and statutory structure ultimately created a program that could not be modified, even when the collective interests of voluntary hospitals demanded it.

Overbuilding increased costs and threatened the viability of existing hospitals to the extent that state and national hospital and Blue Cross associations actively promoted areawide planning. But those hospitals "in line" knew who they were and had an intensely focused interest in avoiding change, while other hospitals were less at risk and therefore less attentive. According to Kenneth Williamson, the AHA's longtime lobbyist, the problem extended even to efforts to secure annual reappropriations from Congress: "That took a lot of work and a lot of support. . . . [b]y and large, the support came from hospitals who hoped to get money from Hill-Burton—some support from those and less support from those who had no interest in it. It was quite a problem."[36]

Because Hill-Burton lacked any strong constituency besides applicant hospitals, Dan Feshbach concludes, state agencies could not mobilize political support for reform and became captives, fearful of provoking controversy.[37] When reforms were made, such as congressional expansion of program benefits to urban hospitals in poor areas, hospital renovation, nursing homes, and community health centers, they were add-ons, written so as to protect the core program's domination by hospitals. Agencies could not shift funds among beneficiary groups, so these reforms failed to induce useful state and local competition between hospitals and other sectors and failed to improve state agencies' bargaining positions vis-à-vis the hospitals.

The Need for More than Capital Funds

The success of Senator Taft's formula for allocating federal funds to states shows that it is possible to achieve an equalization of capital resources by channeling funds from the top down. But Taft's formula did not achieve real redistribution at the intrastate level; well-to-do suburban neighborhoods rather than poor rural areas ultimately received the majority of Hill-Burton's largesse.[38] Hill-Burton required substantial local matching funds before hospitals could be considered for grants, as well as substantial working capital to carry hospitals through the planning stage and into construction (because the first payment was not made until construction actually began).[39] In addition, repeated failures to enact either universal health insurance or public insurance for the elderly and indigent made it very difficult for facilities in poor areas to secure financing and demonstrate financial feasibility—a difficulty they still face today. This combination of rules and environmental conditions made it nearly impossible for many poor communities to benefit from the program. To the extent that future planned payment arrangements seek to promote services not likely to be provided by the competitive market, they will have to provide technical assistance, planning, start-up funds, and probably operating subsidies in addition to capital assistance.

Despite the perverse distributional impact of requiring substantial independent contributions, this provision of the law prevented fly-by-night grantsmanship and—during the period before widespread debt financing and institutional self-sufficiency in fund raising—ensured a degree of real community control, at least at the level of individual and corporate donors. Funds were spent for their intended purpose, as well: they were not moved outside the health system, not misused by applicants, and not invested in institutions that quickly went out of business. This demonstrates the merit of requiring serious real-world tests of managerial capacity and community support before disbursing funds. In new planned payment attempts, when tests based on financial strength or past success would tend to disadvantage the most needy geographic areas or more innovative proposals or sponsors, alternative tests—the equivalent of "sweat equity" in urban housing redevelopment programs—should be devised. New agencies should also be able to reserve funds for applicants who require time to organize themselves or their communities, and should perhaps also be able to disburse funds in stages as such applicants stabilize their support and demonstrate their managerial competence.

Planned Payment Works

Despite the many design shortcomings of the Hill-Burton program, it proved a popular and highly useful program.[40] Compared to the experience of later planning and regulatory programs, it proved that by providing actual funds instead of imposing regulatory restrictions, government can get private institutions to take with enthusiasm actions that they would not otherwise consider. Where Hill-Burton's structure allowed it influence over institutional behavior—in areas related to construction standards rather than community planning or hospital management—the program stimulated cooperative acceptance. As Anne R. Somers remarks, "Hill-Burton architectural, construction, and equipment standards, embodied in national technical guidelines and disseminated primarily through state agency reviews, have had a positive and pervasive influence on the entire hospital industry."[41]

Technical standards undoubtedly increased this influence by telling hospitals exactly what the government wanted them to do. By taking the trouble to write detailed programmatic requirements, Hill-Burton helped assure the behavior it hoped to induce. Similarly, a planned payment system designed, say, to increase community service commitments among HMOs or community hospitals would do well to specify carefully what community services it desires and how it wants them organized. It probably will get greater cooperation in return for its support by taking the trouble to be explicit than by issuing vague statements of objectives or by relying entirely on the goodwill of the institution it supports.[42]

Despite planned payment's moments of impressive success, history also shows how foolhardy it is to attempt to achieve objectives with this mechanism when most of the political and economic forces in the environment push in the opposite direction. The fate of areawide planning in Rochester and in other cities illustrates this nicely. Because the agenda of areawide planners during the 1960s included control of overinvestment and duplicative services, they needed to control almost all sources of capital, which in the long run they lacked the resources to do. A planned payment system operating in a world of economic stringency and limited access to capital might focus instead on filling gaps and preserving selected services. It might not need to control access to capital as much as to have some capital to distribute. But it still would need to set objectives that could coexist with dominant economic incentives and political trends, including a large commercial and for-profit sector and open competition among care management firms.

The history of Hill-Burton's enactment and implementation reinforces this lesson. Good intentions of reformers and legislators cannot compete with the economic and political incentives their actions create; visions of scientific and social progress do not substitute for political economic realities. Reform-minded leaders like Bugbee and Parran proposed, but Congress and later individual hospitals disposed. Public institutions must be in tune with the basic political and economic environment in which they will function; their designers must predict that environment objectively rather than wishfully. Utopian designs mislead, whatever esthetic and consciousness-raising value they may have. A strategic orientation—one that scans the expected environment, clarifies goals, and looks for concrete opportunities to advance them—is more helpful when the time comes to design arrangements that may be implemented.

SUCCESSFUL PLANNED PAYMENT: A BASIC STRUCTURE

U.S. history contains far more proposals to pool capital payment than well-documented examples, and hindsight shows that most of the experiments we know about were imperfectly situated or designed. Nevertheless, it is possible to build on these examples—especially Rochester's 1960–64 fund drive—to describe environments in which planned payment can flourish and program designs that are likely to succeed. A winning combination of environment and mechanism has several key attributes. It would:

- Pool actual funds, place them under the control of a single organization, and give the organization broad discretion to decide how the funds will be spent
- Limit the total funds available from the pool and avoid funding activities that have easy access to alternative sources of funds
- Enable the pool to award funds to several different classes of activity so as to create several competing constituencies
- Separate the top-down allocation of funds to activities from bottom-up evaluation of individual applicants for funds
- Preserve the discretion to shift pooled funds among alternative uses and sectors in response to environmental changes and new priorities
- Avoid an unjustified bias in favor of existing institutions and well-to-do areas by providing operating subsidies as well as capital funds, offering planning and organizing assistance, refraining

from making award decisions on a first-come, first-served basis, and creating provisions for "sweat equity"

- Allocate funds on the basis of their expected ability to advance a predetermined mission, not as entitlements to particular institutions or classes of institutions
- Establish a governance structure for the planned payment organization that is accountable to elected officials and that commands widespread community respect and support
- Avoid creating complex, legalistic rules to govern organizational planning and allocation; encourage negotiation and deliberation with and among recipients of funds; when making grants, seek to approve the best combination of applications rather than review each application sequentially
- Employ qualified managers and analysts in sufficient numbers
- Strike a balance among political accountability, analytic capacity, strategic flexibility, and procedural due process; avoid structural contortions designed to serve one of these objectives at the expense of the others

A planned payment system with these attributes resembles in important respects several other successful institutions that receive and distribute capital funds, including commercial and investment banks, philanthropic foundations, and multi-institutional health services delivery systems. For example, a bank's or a foundation's pool of discretionary funds is limited. This fact both disciplines spending and induces potential recipients of funds to compete and collaborate among themselves, cooperate with the funder's efforts to evaluate their proposals, and work with the bank or foundation over proposal content. Moreover, alternative sources of funds usually are not available. A potential borrower may approach other banks, contact venture capital firms, and consider issuing stock, but all these sources will impose some form of discipline. Economywide, the total pool of available capital is more or less limited, and there are many competitors for access to it. As any academic researcher knows, the sources of grant support for a given research or demonstration projects are even scarcer!

How would a planned payment mechanism with these attributes perform? There is, of course, no analytic method that can answer this question in advance. One way to approach a prediction is to compare such a planned payment mechanism to the major capital regulation program of the recent past, certificate of need. When most people first hear planned payment described, they try to imagine its character and effectiveness by recalling their experience with, or knowledge of, CoN.

Although superficially similar, the two programs in fact differ in fundamental ways. A detailed comparison of CoN and planned payment elucidates these differences and shows why the disappointing CoN experience is a poor predictor of planned payment's potential success.

PLANNED PAYMENT VERSUS CoN

Debate continues over how successful or unsuccessful CoN has been. During an era of nearly unrestrained historical-cost reimbursement, rapid technical change, and general economic inflation and expansion, it is unrealistic to expect CoN to have controlled health care costs by itself.[43] Critics nevertheless often apply this standard of performance.[44] Even using more realistic outcome criteria, however, an airtight evaluation of CoN requires experimentally derived information about what would have happened in the absence of CoN, information we lack. Recent explosions of hospital and nursing home construction following repeal of CoN in some states may provide a sort of natural experiment. They suggest that, absent CoN, cost inflation and excess investment between 1970 and 1985 might have accelerated even more rapidly than they did.[45] Generalizing from such data is difficult, however.

Despite the continuing debate about CoN's effectiveness, the political and administrative history of CoN and "health planning" holds many lessons. Because most of these lessons relate more to regulation and plan writing than to planned payment of capital, to discuss them in further detail would take us off the main path of the argument.[46] It remains important, however, to distinguish clearly between CoN and the kind of planning that accompanied it, on the one hand, and planned payment as it might be implemented, on the other.

How Planned Payment Differs from CoN

A planned payment arrangement that meets the criteria described in the previous section differs fundamentally from certificate of need in several respects.

- CoN awards legal "franchises" to expend capital. Unlike planned payment, CoN does not distribute capital itself. In effect, CoN attempts to tell institutions how they can and cannot spend capital that the institutions regard, of course, as their own.
- The number or long-run incremental costs of the franchises that CoN agencies grant rarely obey any externally imposed aggregate limits, although bed-need formulas and similar standards,

when followed, do represent mechanisms of self-restraint.[47] Planned payment, however, depends on a fund of resources with clear and definite limits.

- CoN attempts to control systemwide capital investment. Although planned payment mechanisms during the era of voluntary areawide planning also had this goal, planned payment need not seek total control to be effective.
- CoN programs usually make decisions on the basis of "black-letter" standards rather than by comparing alternative proposals and alternative combinations of proposals.[48] This legalistic approach—which CoN's regulatory mandate virtually requires—comes at the expense of an ability to operate strategically and opportunistically and to promote extensive negotiation with and among institutions. Although pressures for procedural due process will affect planned payment programs as well, by eschewing a regulatory role and acting like purchasers of services, planned payment programs can more easily promote competition and negotiation and make decisions on the basis of strategy and opportunity rather than fixed rules and standards.
- Finally, the CoN agency waits for applications to appear and must act on applications as it receives them, within a reasonable, often legislatively imposed, period of time. The agency cannot solicit proposals for projects it thinks ought to be undertaken, nor can it provide the developmental and operational support such projects typically need.[49] Planned payment programs can solicit proposals, and they can be organized so as to have funds for start-up costs and operating subsidies as well as for capital support.[50]

Despite the likelihood that CoN imposed a beneficial, constraining influence on investment and cost inflation, students of regulation in general[51] and experts who have studied CoN in detail identify a number of shortcomings. These shortcomings group themselves under three headings: (1) managerial ineffectiveness, (2) passivity, and (3) anticompetitiveness. We review the three with the following question in mind: Can we organize planned payment to avoid these failings?

Managerial Ineffectiveness

Certificate-of-need programs are criticized for staff turnover, inexperienced and inexpert staff, delays, red tape, and other managerial shortcomings. As Penny H. Feldman and Marc J. Roberts[52] and others[53] show in some detail, much of this ineffectiveness can be traced to the inherent political weakness of CoN.

Several aspects of the design of CoN create political weakness. CoN's attentive public consists primarily of hospitals and other potential applicants, often a narrow and highly self-interested group. It is difficult to regulate an industry effectively without countervailing political pressure from sources other than the regulatees.[54] Moreover, CoN franchises are not limited in number, and review is primarily on a first-come, first-served basis. As a result, apart from those who have submitted comparable applications, regulatees within a given industry group lack a strong individual interest to monitor or to influence how other institutions in the group are treated. They have even less interest in the fate of other groups. For the same reasons, provider institutions share little stake in increasing the CoN agency's ability to do its job or in preserving the integrity of the review process. Because, like Hill-Burton, the CoN agency's only true constituency—apart from government—is the recipient institutions, their disinterest and/or active opposition limits the agency's ability to extend its regulatory authority and increase its operating budget.

Lack of funds and authority, in turn, explain much managerial ineffectiveness. Understaffing creates red tape and delay when agencies cannot keep up with the volume of applications. Delay itself becomes a strategy to increase agency negotiating power vis-à-vis applicants. When agency personnel cannot extract useful information from applicants or engage them in constructive bargaining, they also retreat to simple standards and eschew effective, forward planning and negotiation. Simple, rigid review standards also protect beleaguered bureaucrats from additional political controversy, especially charges of favoritism, and provide a natural fortification from which to "hold the line." And it probably is not a coincidence that delay and red tape benefit provider institutions that already own CoN franchises.

To a significant extent, then, structural characteristics of CoN—which planned payment need not share—can be blamed for many of the program's managerial shortcomings. Planned payment, by distributing real resources that institutions want, automatically gains considerable influence and respect. As the areawide planning and Hill-Burton experiences showed, the prospect of gaining access to capital gets everyone's attention and induces a common willingness to take the granting institution's wishes seriously. If, in addition, the pool of funds available for distribution is limited, and other sources of funds for the activity being funded are also limited, each applicant has a greater stake in how other applicants are treated and in the overall integrity of the allocation process. Like the town pump of an earlier era of public health, it will be in all the users' interests to keep planned payment mechanisms clean and flowing. Those who muddy or attempt to divert the flow can expect to be opposed by a larger number committed to protect it.

Planned payment also can be designed to benefit a wider range of interests than CoN. Indeed, as indicated in the previous chapter's mission statement for a capital payment system under competition, an important policy objective for planned payment in the 1990s could be to support public health and community services that a competitive market cannot adequately produce. By creating such a diverse range of potential beneficiaries, planned payment programs can reduce their chance of "capture" by a single narrow constituency. They can "split the opposition," as it were, and make pluralism work for broader objectives in health.

Planned payment programs can further reduce their political vulnerability by periodically reassessing the shares of funds targeted to different programs. This also creates visibility for the planning half of their activity. An actively attended and open planning process, in turn, increases public understanding of the importance of planning to the wider community. This reduces the likelihood that winners or losers will remain unchanged after many cycles of the allocation process.

Despite incentives that favor better management, a planned payment system in a given state could still descend to mediocrity or even to corruption. As the Hill-Burton experience reminds us, the best defense against this possibility is not to displace political and economic competition with a rigid system of rules. Careful crafting of the institution's political and economic structure offers better protection. As we explain in Chapters 4 and 5, design elements such as organizational structure, governing board composition, accountability to governors and legislatures, location in government, multiple beneficiary groups, the creation of targeted subpools of funds, and requirements for public review and participation in agency activities all can improve performance and discourage mediocrity.

For example, an agency organized outside the civil service system might be able to attract better qualified analysts and managers and avoid perpetuating the incentive found in both Hill-Burton and CoN that encourages employees to look forward to eventual employment in the regulated industry. Many of the state agencies and commissions established to provide tax-exempt financing for health care institutions attract and retain able staff. Appendix B describes a planned payment commission operating in the housing industry that also achieves a high standard of managerial competence. Other design elements discussed in Chapters 4 and 5 will be equally healthful, if not more healthful, in their effects.

Passivity

CoN agencies adopt reactive postures in part because that is what they are expected to do and designed to do. Their primary objective is to save money for state Medicaid programs and for other payers by preventing hospitals and other institutions from spending money to acquire and operate programs and facilities.[55] Their legal power is limited to the authority to disapprove attempts to spend money. They are designed to react.

The political impotence previously described further explains the defensive regulatory postures that CoN agencies are apt to adopt. Forced to review applications as they are submitted, limited in their power to negotiate significant project changes, short of staff, time, and money–CoN agencies cannot easily develop or implement aggressive strategic plans based on community needs. Moreover, successful plan development requires more than talent and money; it requires a planning process to which representatives of a broad cross-section of society commit themselves with vigor and responsibility. Participation of this quality does not occur unless it is clear that important decisions ultimately will be taken on the basis of the resulting plan. Yet, as explained above, CoN decisions typically affect only a very narrow group and significantly affect only one or two members within it at any given time. Health planning tied to CoN has never controlled the resources necessary to stimulate a truly active planning process.

Planned payment, on the other hand, can and should be designed to work proactively. Imagine a planned payment system in the 1990s that promotes and finances essential institutions and services that the competitive sector cannot by itself provide. This is a "strategic," interactive role, different from the capital control and rationalization objectives of CoN and some earlier voluntary areawide planning. To the extent that its design and more diverse political constituencies allow it to avoid the passivity of CoN, a new planned payment program can gain the flexibility it needs to act strategically and plan proactively.

Anticompetitiveness

The HMO industry and academic observers have long believed that CoN favors existing institutions and modes of service at the expense of newcomers. The long history of support of CoN by the American Hospital Association, lasting in some states up to the present, reinforces this view in the minds of many. Certainly, the only possible effective way to use CoN to control cost inflation is to limit new investment and prevent expansion of capacity. This capital strangulation strategy, to use

Donald Cohodes's term,[56] clearly favors existing institutions and limits certain forms of competition among them. The strangulation strategy must rely on parallel forms of regulation such as rate setting and licensure for any hope of success; these regulatory cousins also lessen competition.

In the future competitive environment, legislatures and CoN administrators may not continue to pursue a strangulation strategy. If we assume CoN continues after planned payment is introduced—we do not advocate it—then a limited overcapitalization strategy might well be preferable to strangulation. Limited overcapitalization would seek to guarantee enough excess capacity in every locality to facilitate competition without wasting large sums on excessive overbuilding and without losing continuity of service as a result of institutional closure. In addition, with legislative approval, CoN agencies could pursue other social objectives, such as requiring emergency rooms and other essential services to be maintained when renovations are approved.

Some of the historically anticompetitive behavior of CoN programs thus arose from the strangulation tactics they adopted to meet the task and environment they faced. However, the basic structure of CoN programs discourages competition, too. As previously mentioned, agencies rarely limit the aggregate economic value of the franchises they issue, and they must review applications on a first-come, first-served basis. There is thus little competition among their own applicants for the franchises they allocate. In addition, lack of resources and power breed legalism and reliance on rules and standards, which the experienced and well-represented applicant can learn to "game." Alliances with strong, existing providers also become essential to program political survival. All these behaviors discourage competition.

The tradition and assumptions of hierarchical regionalism from which CoN emerged also are essentially anticompetitive. The hierarchal structure of regionalism presupposes a single pyramid in a given geographic area, with technical progress and planning direction flowing from the top down. Such an arrangement may have its benefits, but the promotion of competition is not among them. The bed-need standards and other criteria which CoN programs are legally and administratively bound to use embody the assumptions of regionalism. One difficulty comes when the CoN agency must decide, in an urban or suburban area with several competing institutions, how much of the existing need a particular applicant should be permitted to satisfy. (Alternatively, when there are judged to be excess beds and the agency is reviewing a renovation proposal, it must decide how much of a reduction in the communitywide excess to ask the applicant to accept.) There are only two possible bases for an estimate: the market share the applicant institution already has or the market share the CoN agency thinks it ought to have. Both methods are inherently anticompetitive: they substitute technical opinion for the judgment of the marketplace, and the CoN agency will find little defensible evidence on which to base a decision if it attempts to do anything besides carry forward historical market share.[57] Thus, it is at the level of technical analysis that some of the most anticompetitive effects of CoN are to be found.[58]

Would planned payment be anticompetitive also? There is a tendency to regard CoN as "health planning with teeth" and, to extend the analogy, to imagine planned payment as "CoN with fangs!" Many of the leaders of the old voluntary planning agencies would violently object to the first half of this statement.[59] The half pertaining to planned payment is even less justified. While CoN requires strong rate regulation to succeed in controlling operating costs (and rate regulation requires CoN), planned payment requires neither. Conversely, price competition among hospitals and care management organizations can succeed in controlling costs even when nonmarket institutions are in place to structure market competition and support a cooperative sector. Competitive systems work through incentives, and the incentives introduced by price competition in *operating costs alone* should be more than sufficient to curtail excess utilization and managerial inefficiency (assuming the incentives are "right"). Social allocation of capital, even if extended to the entire hospital industry, could not reverse these powerful incentives on the operating cost side. Indeed, planned capital payment could support competition by providing an antidote to some of the worst side effects of market allocation in health, the sorts of problems highlighted in the Chapter 2 discussion of flat-rate capital payment. HMOs and efficiently managed hospitals will not lose their basic advantage in the marketplace because capital allocation is partly planned.

In the United States, hospital capital needs have been met through a mechanism different than that which provided operating revenues for most of the twentieth century. It was only during the era of historical-cost reimbursement, after the AHA declared that hospitals should be able to meet all financial requirements through cost-based payments, that capital and operating costs were paid identically. The resulting system went rapidly out of control.

Just as we cannot truly measure the impact of CoN in the absence of a well-designed social experiment, it is impossible to gauge the impact of planned payment by comparing it with CoN. What this sort of comparison can establish—quite convincingly—is that planned payment represents a fundamentally different activity than CoN, an activity different in kind rather than degree. Although planned payment obviously gives more real power to communities than CoN ever did, it is entirely wrong to imagine that planned payment would be "that much worse" as a result. As the foregoing comparison indicates, in addition to the other differences between the two activities, planned payment's greater political power and control of resources should make it a much more effective and popular program than CoN.

So far we have discussed planned payment as a generic arrangement, only hinting at how it might be tailored to fit the health system of the 1990s and beyond. We have listed the key structural features that any well-designed planned payment system ought to include, and indicated why they matter. We are now in a position to propose a specific institution. We call it a community health infrastructure bank, or CHIB.

NOTES

1. Victor Rodwin argues in *The Health Planning Predicament* (Berkeley: University of California Press, 1983) that the lack of strong linkages between planning and resource allocation—even in systems Americans imagine are heavily planned like those of Britain and Canada—has neutralized planning's impact. The exception in the United States was described in Chapter 1—the brief "golden age" of voluntary health planning during the middle 1960s when corporate control of philanthropy allowed some cities to achieve encouraging results.
2. To complete the triangle, it is also difficult to discern a link between competent, community-oriented health planning and capital expenditure regulation. Regulation, originally grafted to health planning in the United States to give it "teeth," turns out to be incompatible with planning much of the time. For some of the reasons, see the concluding section of this chapter.
3. I.S. Falk, quoted in Lewis E. Weeks and Howard J. Berman, *Shapers of American Health Care Policy: An Oral History* (Ann Arbor, MI: Health Administration Press, 1985), p. 43.
4. Daniel M. Fox, *Health Policies, Health Politics: The British and American Experience 1911–1965* (Princeton: Princeton University Press, 1986), p. 74. The meaning of this change is ambiguous, since total gross national product dropped over this period.
5. Fox, *Health Policies, Health Politics*, pp. 15–20.
6. Ibid., p. 49.
7. Ibid., p. 93.
8. Marmor makes this point in his study of Medicare's enactment. See Theodore R. Marmor, *The Politics of Medicare* (Hawthorne, NY: Aldine Publishing Co., 1973). So does Daniel M. Fox in *Health Policies, Health Politics*, a recent critique of twentieth-century health care reformers and the historians who chronicle their struggles. In the epilogue to that work, Fox describes Hill-Burton to illustrate how a belief in the inevitable logic and progress of hierarchical regionalism blinded reformers to many of the actual effects of their actions.
9. Richard E. Neustadt, "Presidency and Legislation: The Growth of Central Clearance," *American Political Science Review* 48 (1954): 641–71.
10. George Bugbee, quoted in Weeks and Berman, *Shapers*, p. 36.

11. Maurice Norby, quoted in Weeks and Berman, *Shapers,* pp. 34–35.
12. Ibid., p. 34.
13. Fox, *Health Policies, Health Politics,* p. 123.
14. Bugbee, quoted in Weeks and Berman, *Shapers,* p. 36.
15. Fox, *Health Policies, Health Politics,* p. 126.
16. States were assigned an "allotment percentage" that equaled 1.00 minus .50 (state per capita income/U.S. per capita income), but not less than .33 or more than .75. This percentage times the state's population, divided by analogous figures for all other states and multiplied by the annual federal appropriation, gave the state's share. P.L. 79-725, Sec. 631 (a).
17. "The fellow whose ingenuity made that formula possible was a member of my staff named Daniel Gerig. I never forget to give him credit for it." Neither shall we. I.S. Falk, quoted in Weeks and Berman, *Shapers,* p. 42.
18. Fox, *Health Policies, Health Politics,* p. 130.
19. Judith Lave and Lester Lave, *The Hospital Construction Act: An Evaluation of the Hill-Burton Program, 1948–1973* (Washington, DC: American Enterprise Institute for Public Policy Research, 1974).
20. Exactly this dynamic appears in attempts by the Commonwealth Fund and other foundations to support hospital construction and community health planning in rural areas during the 1930s and 1940s. See Peter Buck, "Why Not the Best? Some Reasons and Examples from Child Health and Rural Hospitals," *Journal of Social History* 18: (1985): 413–31.
21. For a description of one such effort, see Walter J. McNerny, *Hospital and Medical Economics* (Chicago: Hospital Research and Educational Trust, 1962), p. 1382; see also Walter J. McNerny and Donald C. Riedel, *Regionalization and Rural Health Care: An Experiment in Three Communities* (Ann Arbor, MI: University of Michigan Press, 1962).
22. In one upstate New York area, three new, underutilized hospitals were built in close proximity to one another because the state facility plan measured bed need by county, and each of the hospitals was located in a separate county. See Jonathan B. Brown, *Facility Expansion and Facility Closure: Two Case Studies in Health Planning and Regulation from Rochester, New York* (Boston: Center for Community Health and Medical Care, Harvard University 1978).
23. Anne R. Somers, *Hospital Regulation: The Dilemma of Public Policy* (Princeton: Industrial Relations Section, Princeton University, 1969).
24. Somers, *Hospital Regulation,* p. 138.
25. Symond R. Gottlieb, "A Brief History of Health Planning in the United States." In Clark R. Havighurst, ed., *Regulating Health Facilities Construction* (Washington, DC: American Enterprise Institute, 1974), p. 15.
26. Theodore R. Marmor and James A. Morone, "Representing Consumer Interests: Imbalanced Markets, Health Planning, and the HSAs," *Milbank Memorial Fund Quarterly/Health and Society* 3 (1984): 85; Bruce C. Vladeck, "Interest Group Representation and the HSAs: Health Planning and Political Theory," *American Journal of Public Health* 67 (1977): 223–29.
27. Public Law 79-725, Sec. 635.
28. Truman saw this as an especially dangerous precedent and came close to vetoing the bill on that account. Bugbee was not invited to the signing because he had pressed so hard to give the council its regulatory powers. See Weeks and Berman, *Shapers,* p. 48.
29. States later were given discretion to raise the percentage of support to 67

percent and to vary it among applicants. Apparently, no state elected to provide more than 50 percent financing. I.S. Falk, quoted in Weeks and Berman, *Shapers*, p. 43.

30. *Code of Federal Regulations*, 1949, Title 42, Ch. 1, Part 53, pp. 167ff.
31. Dan Feshbach, "What's Inside the Black Box: A Case Study of Allocative Politics in the Hill-Burton Program," *International Journal of Health Services* 9 (1979): 325.
32. Brown, *Facility Expansion*.
33. Feshbach, "What's Inside the Black Box."
34. Ibid.
35. Commission on Hospital Care, *Hospital Care in the United States* (New York: Commonwealth Fund, 1947), "Introductory Statement," reprinted in Weeks and Berman, *Shapers*, pp. 277–79.
36. Kenneth Williamson, chief lobbyist for the American Hospital Association from 1954 to 1972, quoted in Weeks and Berman, *Shapers*, p. 212.
37. Feshbach, "What's Inside the Black Box."
38. Ibid.
39. Ibid., p. 326.
40. Somers, *Hospital Regulation*, p. 135.
41. Ibid.
42. Robert M. Sigmond, "Re-Examining the Role of the Community Hospital in a Competitive Environment," The Michael M. Davis Lecture, Center for Health Administration Studies, University of Chicago, 1985.
43. Committee on Health Planning Goals and Standards, Institute of Medicine, *Health Planning in the United States* (Washington, DC: National Academy Press, 1981).
44. Paul L. Joskow, *Controlling Hospital Costs* (Cambridge, MA: MIT Press, 1980); Policy Analysis, Inc. *Evaluation of the Effects of Certificate-of-Need Programs, Final Report* (Boston: Policy Analysis, Inc., 1980).
45. James B. Simpson, "State Certificate of Need Programs: The Current Status," *American Journal of Public Health* 75 (1985): 1225–29.
46. A number of excellent accounts are available. See, for example, Committee on Health Planning Goals and Standards, *Health Planning in the United States*; Bonnie Lefcowitz, *Health Planning: Lessons for the Future* (Rockville, MD: Aspen Systems Corporation, 1983); Drew Altman, Richard Greene, and Harvey M. Sapolsky, *Health Planning and Regulation: The Decision-Making Process* (Washington, DC and Ann Arbor, MI: AUPHA Press, 1981).
47. One of the first evaluations of CoN suggested that hospitals subject to CoN substituted investments in equipment and technology which were not subject to CoN review for investments in beds and plant that they otherwise might have made. See David Salkever and Thomas Bice, "The Impact of Certificate-of-Need Controls on Hospital Investment," *Milbank Memorial Fund Quarterly* 54 (1976): 185–214.
48. Some states have tried to batch CoN applications in an attempt to introduce competition and comparison shopping into their reviews. Annual caps on the incremental cost of approved projects also have this objective. For a discussion of "capital caps," see Wendy M. Greenfield, "New Approaches to Using the Determination of Need Process to Contain Hospital Costs," *New England Journal of Medicine* 309 (1983): 372–74; Carol V. Getts, *Methods for Establishing Capital Expenditure Limits* (Madison, WI: Institute for Health

Planning, 1984); ICF, Inc., *An Analysis of Programs to Limit Hospital Expenditures. Final Report*. (Washington, DC: ICF, Inc., 1980).

49. If delivery organizations are not addressing community needs, it usually is because they cannot break even doing so or because other investment opportunities are more remunerative.
50. Some CoN programs—those located in the few states with global-budget, revenue-cap, hospital cost control systems—could control the incremental operating costs of the capital projects they approved through agreements with the rate-setting agencies. The control was a negative one, limited to services already being reimbursed and, usually, to projects sponsored by hospitals.
51. See, for example, Stephen Breyer, *Regulation and Its Reform* (Cambridge, MA: Harvard University Press, 1982).
52. Penny H. Feldman and Marc J. Roberts, "Magic Bullets or Seven-Card Stud: Understanding Health Care Regulation." In R. Gordon, ed., *Issues in Health Care Regulation* (New York: McGraw-Hill, 1980).
53. Altman, Greene, and Sapolsky, *Health Planning and Regulation*.
54. Theodore R. Marmor and James A. Morone, "Representing Consumer Interests: Imbalanced Markets, Health Planning, and the HSAs," *Milbank Memorial Fund Quarterly* 58 (1980): 125–65; Vladeck, "Interest Group Representation and the HSAs; E.E. Schattschneider, *The Semi-Sovereign People: A Realist's View of Democracy in America* (New York: Holt, Rinehart & Winston, 1960).
55. CoN programs can also serve important quality and access promotion functions, as when they maintain the caseloads and hence the quality of cardiac surgical programs by limiting market entry. Access and program design conditions also may be attached to CoN approvals. These are not the essential functions of CoN, however, and both of them could equally well be carried out by a properly designed licensure program.
56. Donald Cohodes, "The View from the States." In Office for Health Facilities, Health Resources Administration, U.S. Department of Health and Human Services, *Health Capital Issues* (Washington, DC: U.S. Government Printing Office, 1983).
57. The Appropriateness Evaluation Protocol has been used in Massachusetts starting in 1986 to create an exception to the bed need formula for institutions that appear exceptionally well managed in terms of unnecessary admissions and bed days. So far, use of this instrument has been controversial. See Paul M. Gertman and Joseph D. Restuccia, "The Appropriateness Evaluation Protocol: A Technique for Assessing Unnecessary Days of Hospital Care," *Medical Care* 19 (August 1981): 855; Joseph D. Restuccia, Paul M. Gertman, and Susan J. Dayno, *Methods to Determine Inappropriate Use of Hospital Resources: Final Report* (Boston: Health Care Research Unit, Boston University Medical Center, 1982).
58. Stephen Breyer described a similar regulatory conundrum known as the allocation of "joint costs" in *Regulation*, pp. 55–56.
59. Consider the quotation from Sieverts presented in Chapter 1, or this statement by Anne R. Somers in *Hospital Regulation*, p. 141: "One of the striking facts about voluntary bodies is that many of them do not want responsibility for real decision-making. The reasoning behind this view is not usually laziness or irresponsibility on the part of the planners but a well-founded opposition to any attempt to impose some arbitrary 'master plan' on a com-

munity, appreciation of the fact that creative hospital planning should usually start with the individual institution, and a commendable modesty with respect to present planning techniques and methodology."

4.

The Community Health Infrastructure Bank: A Proposal

Jonathan B. Brown with contributions by *Stephen R. Thomas* and *David W. Young*

The idea of pooling resources and then reallocating them to health care institutions on the basis of need, merit, or other criteria arises frequently these days. Several states divert a percentage of hospital reimbursement or tax hospital revenues to create "bad debt and free care pools" to subsidize the operations of hospitals serving the poor.[1] In 1986, Congress came very close to imposing caps on the annual dollar value of tax-exempt debt that any state could issue for hospitals and other health care institutions. Such caps would have created a limited annual pool of tax-exempt financing; states would have had to develop plans or criteria to govern allocation of the funds.[2] Many of the state agencies that issue tax-exempt hospital bonds also have created "blind equipment pools"—bond offerings that generate a limited fund from which participating hospitals may borrow as needed for small-ticket capital needs.[3] The state of New York recently asked the federal Health Care Financing Administration for a waiver of Medicare's payment rules to establish a pool of a different kind, one that would capture the federal payments for medical education costs that now go directly to hospitals. The state would then redistribute these funds to institutions according to the need for residencies in various specialties, hospitals, neighborhoods, and communities. The nation's public hospitals have requested the enactment of a federal program to subsidize the capital needs of institutions that serve disproportionate numbers of poor and uninsured patients. Like Hill-Burton, such a program would create a kind of planned payment system for capital.

Perhaps the most advanced example of a capital pool has been operating in Rochester, New York since 1980. In that year, Rochester's nine hospitals created the Hospital Experimental Payment program, known as HEP. They agreed among themselves to ask private and governmental payers to limit all the community's payments for hospital services to a preset annual amount, which the hospitals would then pool and allocate among themselves. They also agreed to use these funds to establish several special pools, including one to finance nonroutine capital expenditures. In 1985, the hospitals extended their contract and amended the program's design to include a communitywide cap on capital expenditures. Stephen R. Thomas studied the Rochester pooling system in detail on behalf of the Health Capital Project; his report and evaluation of how community capital decisions are made within this system appear in Appendix A. The experiment appears quite successful, although the willingness of the member hospitals to continue it depends on changes in the state and national hospital reimbursement environment which could make continued pooling unattractive.

What sort of systemwide planned capital payment or pooling mechanism would work in U.S. communities in the years to come? In Chapter 2 we identified six basic objectives appropriate to the emerging competitive environment:

1. Maintain an accessible and efficient capital infrastructure and preserve society's investment in health capital.
2. Launch and support essential services that existing markets cannot supply.
3. Identify and strengthen a cooperative sector within the health services industry.
4. Stimulate experimentation and innovation in the organization and delivery of service.
5. Strengthen and broaden community capacity to plan and act.
6. Preserve and promote effective competitive markets.

In addition, in Chapter 3 we used the history of earlier planned payment attempts to identify what it takes to make planned payment work well. These lessons boil down to seven basic design rules:

1. Pool actual funds, not franchises or licenses to use funds.
2. Limit the size of the pool.
3. Create competing constituencies by allocating funds to several health industry sectors.

4. Provide funds for organizing, planning, and operating subsidies as well as for capital; allow applicants to contribute sweat equity as well as financial equity.
5. Create a single organization to manage the funds, and let it shift funds among sectors; make it accountable to the community both through elected officials and through nongovernmental community leaders.
6. Have the organization make allocational decisions on the basis of outcome-oriented strategic plans and negotiations with applicants; avoid legalistic decision rules and first-come first-served review processes.
7. Give the organization adequate operating funds to hire sufficient numbers of qualified managers, analysts, and organizers.

In this chapter we propose a specific institution, called a community health infrastructure bank, that unites these seven design rules with the six basic objectives summarized above. We consider how such a bank should be designed in terms of its coverage, its sources of funds, the forms in which it distributes funds, its planning and management systems, and its organizational structure. In Chapter 5, we analyze in detail how the bank—or CHIB—ought to be governed and where it should locate in relation to existing governmental and private institutions.

COVERAGE

A fundamental early decision in the design of any planned payment program is its "coverage"—the number of health system "sectors" and, within sectors, the proportion of service delivery institutions that the program will help support. For example, the Rochester HEP program could be said to exhibit a moderate degree of coverage. HEP pools capital and operating funds (including a fund to cover bad debt and charity expenses) for all of Rochester's hospitals; however, it does not allocate funds to nonhospital sectors, such as long-term care, environmental health, medical education, research, or primary care, except to the extent that hospitals provide such services.

The discussions in the preceding chapter of Hill-Burton and certificate of need indicate that broad, multisectoral coverage helps planned payment programs avoid capture by beneficiary groups. Broad coverage also stimulates competition among beneficiaries, leading to better data, more effective planning, and better award decisions. Thus, a robust CHIB design will include *broad coverage*.

The CHIB mission also requires broad, multisectoral coverage. This mission seeks to define and support a cooperative sector that cuts across traditional industry groupings, promotes innovation in the design of services and institutions, and rescues and redistributes some of the excess capital that has accumulated in the acute care hospital sector. This mission requires the CHIB to support several institutional types. In addition, as traditional industry sectors like insurance, hospital care, long-term care, benefits management, and ambulatory care merge and mutate, it would be difficult for any planned payment system to focus on one or two current institutional types and expect to remain relevant for very long.

Within industry sectors, history shows that the planned payment systems of the past—Hill-Burton and voluntary areawide planning—lost effectiveness when they were not the dominant source of financing for the activities they sought to support.[4] Hill-Burton, for example, could not induce multi-institutional coordination or limit beds per capita when 70 percent of construction did not use Hill-Burton support. The CHIB mission, in part, is to establish a cooperative sector; commercially oriented hospitals and other institutions will continue to compete in a more open market. Therefore, the CHIB need not, indeed should not, control resources used by all institutions, systemwide. However, *within the cooperative sector* a CHIB will need to control enough of the resources available to particular institutions to ensure that they act cooperatively in return for community support.

To carry this degree of influence, a CHIB need not control all the capital and operating revenues of cooperative-sector institutions. As Chapter 1 makes plain, most of the revenues of health services delivery organizations are not discretionary; they support ongoing, day-to-day operations. This is why discretionary funds exert a far greater influence on organizational behavior than their relative dollar value might indicate. The potential of small streams of money is illustrated by the eagerness with which many voluntary hospitals join national chains and alliances to increase their access to capital, and by the fact that "capital" reimbursement makes the difference between solvency and bankruptcy on occasion for many hospitals. Discretionary funds determine an institution's ability to restore itself, to evolve, and ultimately to survive. By controlling a large portion of *discretionary* resources in the cooperative sector, CHIBs should be able to exert substantial leverage over institutional behavior and, in the long run, over organizational values and culture.

The CHIB's mission is to *provide* capital and support essential services in institutions that cannot get the resources elsewhere, not to *control* capital investment systemwide. By definition, such a mission guarantees that CHIBs will control the lion's share of the funds that are available to support the services it wants to support. Services that enjoy other forms of support would not be candidates for CHIB support. In a competitive health care environment, commercial sources will provide few funds for community services. A CHIB with goals like those we propose will neither need nor want to support community services that the market does provide.

If difficulties arise in the match between CHIB coverage and mission, they may occur when a CHIB tries to fund a limited package of community-oriented services in a well-capitalized, financially secure, commercially oriented institution. Imagine, for example, a state in which the managed care market became dominated by a few for-profit managed care corporations that made adequate profits and consequently enjoyed ready access to capital. A CHIB might request each of these HMOs to take epidemiologic responsibility for the population of a given geographic area and ask them to cooperate with each other in providing community-oriented services to residents. But only a minority of residents in any particular catchment area would be involved in the HMO with responsibility for that area, so each HMO would capture only a minority of the health benefits its community activities generated. It would also have to develop a new administrative unit to deliver the community services, as it would not see most community members in the normal course of ambulatory care.

In this situation, both the corporate culture of the HMOs and their competitiveness might make it difficult for them to do what the CHIB requested. Their controlling incentives would be antagonistic to the CHIB's objectives, and the CHIB would not contribute sufficient resources to change those incentives. Moreover, since one of the CHIB's objectives is to preserve competition where it works well, it would not want to change the dominant incentives anyway. Problems like this arose during the 1960s and early 1970s when the federal government tried to get major urban teaching hospitals to establish community-oriented and community-*controlled* neighborhood health centers. The resulting clash of culture and interests greatly reduced the neighborhood health center program's effectiveness in some areas. The CHIB's solution in situations such as this is to avoid launching programs that its coverage is too narrow to implement. There will be many such situations.

A second form of inadequate coverage could arise if two or more governmental and philanthropic programs sought to address a particular community's needs in contradictory ways. For example, if a CHIB were established without repealing CoN review for institutions the CHIB supported, conflicting decisions might occur. A state that decides to create a CHIB will need to review carefully potential problems of intergovernmental coordination.[5]

SOURCES OF FUNDS

A CHIB established by a state legislature can be funded from up to five basic sources:

- New taxes
- Diversions from the revenues of provider institutions or insurers
- Federal block grant funds
- Appropriations from existing general revenues
- Philanthropy

In addition, control over access to tax-exempt debt for health care institutions could be transferred to the CHIB.

How Much Funding is Needed?

The amount of funding required from these sources will depend on the precise mission the legislature (or other sponsoring organization) envisions for the CHIB, as well as on local economic and social conditions. To focus for the moment on the hospital sector, imagine a rural state in which hospitals are widely distributed, isolated, and small; a large percentage of them, therefore, may both provide essential community services not available elsewhere and face financial difficulty because they cannot take advantage of economies of scale. Such a state might need to provide long-run capital support for most of its hospitals and would require a relatively large pool of funds to do so. A similar situation might prevail in an urban state with an oversupply of beds but only a few major hospitals in poor neighborhoods, hospitals that have not been able to rebuild and stay abreast of technologic change. A fairly large near-term investment in such hospitals might be required–and therefore a fairly large pool of CHIB resources–even though the state's hospital infrastructure on the whole is both modern and overbedded.

Each state or region will have to project its CHIB's income requirements carefully. Looking still at acute hospital plant and fixed equipment ("big-ticket") costs, only, the largest stream of funds that any CHIB would need probably would not exceed the flow of funds that currently enters the acute care sector as reimbursement for big-ticket expenditures. In recent years, the explicit capital reimbursement that Medicare pays U.S. hospitals has totaled between 7 percent and 8 percent of the hospitals' annual operating cost reimbursement. The amount attributable to big-ticket capital costs—construction and fixed equipment—is about 5 percent; roughly one-third of this amount goes for interest payments.[6] In hospitals that have recently rebuilt or expanded, total capital reimbursement as a percentage of operating reimbursement is much higher—more than 10 percent, sometimes 20 percent or more.[7] However, for each such high-percentage hospital, there are several hospitals in the later stages of their capital cycles with percentages below the average.

Annual payments are higher to hospitals with new construction for two reasons. First, due to inflation, replacement cost exceeds the original historical cost of any facility being replaced. Thus, the depreciation payments hospitals receive for older buildings are less than the depreciation payments Medicare (which calculates depreciation on the basis of historical costs) makes for new ones. Second, early payments to bondholders consist almost entirely of payments on current and future interest, which Medicare reimburses in full in addition to paying for straight-line depreciation based on the cost of the new plant. Thus, some of the jump in capital-related reimbursement for new facilities reflects the truly higher cost of replacement, and some may be considered an artifact of debt financing, financial conventions, and reimbursement rules. Depending on the forms in which a CHIB disburses funds (grants versus loans, for example), it could cut its revenue needs well below comparable cost-based reimbursement levels.

A CHIB could further reduce its costs by not rebuilding more excess beds than are needed to preserve competition, and by building less extravagant institutions than cost-based reimbursement encouraged in the past. Contributions from other sources—internal reserves and future surpluses, the hospital's medical staff, philanthropy—could further reduce funding needs. A CHIB in a state with a low proportion of financially distressed, essential institutions could, of course, maintain hospital infrastructure with even fewer resources.

Hospital renovation and replacement are not the sole end-uses for CHIB funds. Significant additional funds could be allocated to support community-oriented activity in other sectors—long-term care, primary care, mental health, environmental health—and for activities of community importance that cut across these sectors—education, disease prevention, research, indigent care, community organizing, and perhaps others. (Thus the term *infrastructure* in community health infrastructure bank refers to several kinds of community capital: physical capital, technical capital, human capital, programmatic capital, and cultural capital.) Each state that considers creating a CHIB will need to estimate its CHIB's revenue needs in light of the mission it gives the CHIB and the characteristics of its health system. In the case of hospital construction needs, the state will also need to consider the timing of anticipated needs. Major replacement projects are both massive and relatively infrequent, and they often arise in expensive clusters.

Where Should Funds Come From?

Hospital renovation and replacement, alone, represent very significant expenditures. Estimates of annual hospital construction needs for the next decade (1986–95) range between roughly $7 billion to $46 billion per year for the nation as a whole.[8] The lower end of this range appears more realistic, however.[9] Taking $10 billion per year as a base figure and assuming that, at a minimum, 25 percent of future construction would be in hospitals meriting CHIB support, revenues on the order of $2.5 billion would be needed each year simply to fund the big-ticket hospital construction activities of U.S. CHIBs, if there were a CHIB in every state. Yet, the huge federal deficit and the constraints on existing revenues in many states limit the amount of funds that they can appropriate without new taxes. Some states might be both able and willing to fund hospital construction needs in the community-oriented sector from existing tax revenues, but we expect that in most states either new taxes or some arrangement to divert funds from the existing health services reimbursement stream will be more palatable. Each state's choice between the latter two options will require detailed study and will depend on its particular circumstances and politics. In this presentation, we can only review some of the options and considerations that states should take into account.

A tax on wages. Presumably, a new tax would take the form of a tax either on the wages or on the health benefit payments paid by employers. A tax on wages would tend to equalize the burden of contribution borne by larger firms, which typically offer generous health insurance benefits, with that borne by smaller firms, which typically do not. To the extent that the lack of health insurance among employed persons is one of the fundamental reasons why an exclusively competitive health care system cannot meet community needs, there is a certain fairness to this approach. Even if nominally paid by employers, however, such a tax would come at least in part from employee earnings because employers would recoup all or part of the cost in the long run in the form of lower wage payments. As with social security, direct contributions from employees might even be required. A flat-rate tax on wages would therefore be regressive; it would take a larger proportion of income from low-wage employees than from high-wage earners unless the marginal tax rate were made to vary with annual wages.

But tinkering of that sort gets complicated. Does one ignore the differences in income between families with one wage earner and families with more than one wage earner? Should the tax rate vary with family size? What about part-time workers and workers with two jobs? Any tax sophisticated enough to be nonregressive quickly starts to resemble an income tax in terms of the information and paperwork required to administer it. In states that already collect a progressive or proportional state income tax, an additional tax on wages could be grafted to existing reporting and collection mechanisms. But such a tax would become primarily a tax on individual incomes, because it no longer would be collected from employers. And a change in income taxation is a major political act, one not likely to be taken simply to fund a CHIB. To keep personal, after-tax income from dropping precipitously, and to avoid the politics of income taxation, it may be necessary to look to employers for tax revenues—if the CHIB is to be financed by taxes—and to accept the attendant regressivity and insensitivity that taxing employers brings.

Is the price of regressivity worth paying to force businesses that do not now offer adequate health insurance to bear some of the costs? Alternative policies are available to make this happen, after all—state legislatures could simply require employers to provide health insurance and could develop programs to give small firms some of the large-group discounts that major firms now enjoy. In states that adopt a tax on wages to support a pool to pay for the costs of indigent care (which a CHIB might be asked to allocate), then the use of a wage tax to finance other CHIB activities might be practical. Otherwise, collection costs and the regressivity of the arrangement do not seem worth incurring.

A diversion of health insurance premiums. A diversion from health insurance premiums differs from a wage tax in important respects. It fails to equalize the incidence of taxation between employers who offer health insurance and those who do not, because employers that do not offer health insurance avoid the diversion. It does offer other advantages, however. One is that there are far fewer health insurance firms than employers. If the tax were collected from insurers and other fiscal intermediaries, the collection process would be simplified and collection costs reduced. Intermediaries, in turn, would pass the cost of the tax back to employers, unions, and individual purchasers of health insurance in the form of higher premiums. If collected from insurers rather than employers, a tax on health insurance premiums would also keep the collection of revenues within the health care system. It represents more a diversion or reallocation of resources than a tax. As such, it might cause fewer political problems for governors and legislative leaders.

Many reformers also believe that taxation of health benefits will encourage more efficient consumer use of health services and, ultimately, a more efficient health care system. They argue that taxing premiums will encourage more careful shopping by consumers because it equalizes the trade-off between money wages and employer contributions to health insurance premiums. Price-conscious consumers, in turn, will encourage the development of less expensive health insurance plans and of plans that require greater out-of-pocket participation from enrollees.[10] Or so the argument goes. Empirical data do not seem to support the notion that greater cost sharing by employees lowers prices and increases competition.[11] And the tax itself would be regressive, since the increased cost of health insurance, when and *if* translated into greater out-of-pocket cost sharing by employees, would consume a greater share of the wages of low-income employees.[12] Still, many people support the idea because of these predicted incentive effects.

Diverting a portion of the revenues that flow to insurers and related firms, though far simpler than a tax on wages or incomes, still requires sophisticated implementation. New organizational forms are appearing at a dizzying rate–organizations that combine insurance, brokering, contracting, and service delivery functions. In addition, most large corporations no longer pay state taxes on insurance premiums because they self-insure, using insurance companies to provide "administrative services only" (ASO). The state would have to locate and intercept funds whenever they move from the original purchaser of services–an individual or an employer or a union trust fund–to any of a variety of organizations. The state must divert a percentage of the total health care–related premium receipts of Blue Cross and commercial insurance plans, of HMOs, and of any other organizations that provide insurance as part of the service they sell. In addition, it must tax the receipts of any ASO or health benefits brokering organization. Finally, it must tax any revenues of health care providers–possibly including physicians and other group and solo practitioners with receipts above a certain threshold–that do not pass through the hands of one of the above-listed intermediaries. In the case of direct fee-for-service and contract payments to providers, it might be simpler and less controversial to tax directly the few self-insuring employers who do not use ASO intermediaries.

These arrangements would apply to payments made to private fiscal intermediaries. It is not possible for a state to tax the revenues of Medicare. Similarly, a mechanism to make contributions on behalf of the state's own Medicaid program would have to be devised. The anticipated shift to prospective capital payment by Medicare and by many state Medicaid programs will facilitate diversion, however. In the case of Medicare, states can apply to HCFA for waivers that will permit them to assume control of a portion of the payments earmarked for the capital requirements of hospitals.[13] Diversion of federal payments to other providers, such as physicians, would be more difficult to implement.

A diversion of provider revenues. The third basic financing option for major CHIB expenditures is to divert funds from the revenues of providers of direct care. New York, New Jersey, Maryland, and Massachusetts, states that sequester a portion of hospital reimbursement to pay for the costs of bad debt and free care, do this already. This also is how the Rochester hospital experimental payment program creates its pools for capital, bad debt, and innovation. Florida currently taxes hospital revenues to provide a pool of funds to support indigent care.

Diversion from providers shares some of the political advantages of taxation of health insurance and related receipts, in that it keeps the diversion process within the health care system. It also allows the state to maintain a more direct relationship between the industry groups that receive CHIB funds and the groups that provide them. Thus, acute care hospitals would both contribute and receive funds; the commercial stratum within a given industry sector would contribute to the community stratum within the same sector. The CHIB would be free to redistribute funds among sectors—a freedom essential to its mission but there would remain an observable relationship between donors and recipients.

It is reasonable to ask the commercial stratum to subsidize the community stratum within an industry. Most of the payments accepted by all providers are, after all, social funds. About half come from taxation through Medicare and Medicaid. Much of the remainder are raised by Blue Cross plans which are chartered by state legislatures as non-profit, community payment mechanisms and, until 1986, also were exempt from federal taxation. Even the commercial insurance companies enjoy immunity from antitrust laws and function (in their insurance role) as bookkeepers and poolers of risk for purchasers of services—a social function—not as producers of services.

Moreover, commercially oriented hospitals and other providers benefit from the existence of community-oriented hospitals willing to serve the poor and provide unprofitable services. The cooperative sector treats patients that the competitive sector would otherwise be under pressure to accept on a charity basis. Preventive and environmental services similarly reduce the cost of coverage for insurance companies and health maintenance organizations. In addition, a strong cooperative sector reduces political pressure to decommercialize the entire health care system, thereby permitting commercial institutions to go about their business with less threat of interference. A commercial sector that benefits so much from community-oriented institutions should pay a large share toward supporting them.

The diversion of funds from direct providers of service would be reasonably simple to implement, compared to the health insurance premium taxation arrangements previously discussed. Prospective capital payment by Medicare will facilitate the diversion of federal revenues by removing implied institutional entitlements to payment and isolating capital payments in a separate stream. Care will have to be taken to identify all providers of services and their revenues, though. Many hospitals in "regulated states" such as New York[14] and Massachusetts[15] changed their corporate structure to insulate portions of their revenues from rate-setting controls in recent years, as have hospitals in other states for tax and entrepreneurial reasons. Payments for hospitalization and other services may be buried among the internal transactions of such vertically and horizontally integrated corporate providers. The books of national firms would probably have to be scrutinized with particular care, since some of their revenues will come from national accounts to cover care delivered, but not paid for, in the state where the CHIB is to be located.

To the extent that diversions from the revenues of commercially oriented delivery institutions result in increased prices to buyers of services, and to the extent that employers and union trust funds pass these price increases on to employees in the form of increased out-of-pocket payments or decreased coverage, then the diversion of funds from provider revenues will create a regressive tax on lower-income employees. As we have seen, though, this is true of all financing options except appropriations from general revenues in the very few states with progressive income taxes. At least, in the case of diversions from provider revenues, the regressive impact is likely to become highly attenuated by the time it reaches the individual employee. Diversion of provider revenues also gives states a chance to expand or contract a CHIB's coverage for substantive policy reasons without having to raise or lower general purpose taxes to do it. New industry sectors can be brought in or out as appropriate without affecting the participation of other sectors or altering the tax rates faced by individuals or employers.

It should be noted that most of the current hospital capital reimbursement stream is implicitly committed to the retirement of existing debt. Although most cost-based payers do not reimburse directly for the retirement of debt principal, they pay for interest expense and they reimburse depreciation costs. Many hospitals rely on these depreciation and interest payments to repay bondholders and other lenders. In the future, they will rely on flat-rate capital payments. Therefore, only a small percentage of the hospital capital payment stream can realistically be considered available for diversion to the CHIB's account on the day a CHIB is established, unless a state hopes to abruptly squeeze a great deal more "fat" from the system than seems likely.[16] A gradual increase of the CHIB's diversion rate – akin to the blending formulas proposed by designers of flat-rate capital payment systems – therefore will be necessary. The process might be more effective than blending in the flat-rate case because the CHIB would have responsibility for the survival of those institutions in financial distress that were deemed essential providers, and so could mitigate any adverse effects of the formulaic approach.

Note that rates of growth in aggregate institutional reimbursement will affect the degree of hardship caused by the rising proportion of funds diverted to the CHIB: when inflation in medical costs is high, existing indebtedness as a proportion of total revenues drops and it is easier to repay. The size of the CHIB's diversion rate also will exert a strong effect on the number of hospitals and other providers that come to depend on it for capital and operating support. A higher diversion rate will decrease institutional revenues to a greater extent so that, although the CHIB has more funds in its pool, there will be more institutions in financial distress to make a claim on its resources. Detailed analysis in a particular state may reveal a crossover point at which additional diversions are counterproductive. To repeat, the final decision about how many institutions to support, and how much funding to provide the CHIB, should be derived from a careful identification of local needs and resources.

Block Grant Funds and General Revenue Appropriations

A state legislature could also appropriate general revenue funds to support CHIB activities, and it could place federal block grant funds under the CHIB's control. These sources of funds, while not likely to be large enough to finance more than a portion of big-ticket hospital construction in a state, could be used to support and capitalize health centers, to fund environmental programs, for technical support and start-up funds, and for many other, lower-cost purposes. In appropriating such funds to the CHIB's use, however, legislatures should take care not to limit narrowly the purposes for which they may be used. As previously discussed, it will be essential to CHIB success that a capacity to move funds freely among purposes, regions, and institutional sectors be preserved. When this flexibility is missing, focused institutional interests can more easily "capture" the CHIB's planning and administrative structure, and the capacity to plan strategically will be lost. Lack of flexibility may be especially troublesome in the case of narrowly targetted health block grant funds. One federal block grant, for example, is intended solely for the support of community health centers. Unless the CHIB wanted to allocate considerable additional moneys to health centers from its discretionary funds, or change radically the shares that individual health centers receive, a legislature probably should not ask the CHIB to distribute this dedicated block grant.

Access to Tax-Exempt Debt

Although not a pool of funds directly under CHIB control, the tax-exempt debt that state health facility finance agencies provide represents a source of capital that should be conditioned on community service, if only to justify its exemption from taxation.[17] Congress in 1986 came close to limiting by state the total annual borrowing hospitals could undertake in the tax-exempt market; it did limit tax-exempt borrowing by many other users. Thus, tax-exempt debt may in the future begin to resemble the *limited* pool of resources that is essential to any CHIB. Moreover, any CHIB that seeks to define and support a community sector within the health care system probably needs to control, for planning purposes, as much as possible of the discretionary capital and operating resources earmarked for community service institutions. Problems of interagency coordination would also be avoided by placing tax-exempt bonding within the CHIB's mandate.

Many state health facilities financing authorities have achieved impressive levels of expertise. Some of them offer models for CHIBs to emulate in terms of governance structure and staff effectiveness. Legislatures in some states might opt to use the local authority as the base on which to build a CHIB. Alternatively, legislators could transfer the legal authority to issue new tax-exempt debt to a newly created CHIB. The choice might turn on the organizational culture of the financing authority. If it is very passive—seeing itself as simply a conduit between hospitals and the debt market, as many financing authorities do—the legislature might be wise to look elsewhere for more active leadership.

Philanthropy

Prior to the great expansion of governmental activity during the New Deal and World War II, it was common for philanthropists to donate substantial funds to the government. When C. Rufus Rorem wrote about "the public's investment in hospitals" in 1930, that public investment was derived from the contributions of individual donors, not government. It is not impossible to imagine private persons contributing funds to a CHIB located in state government. At a minimum, CHIBs could try to coordinate their giving with local hospital funds and United Way agencies.

In the hospital sector, the long-term decline in philanthropic support is undoubtedly due in part to a correct perception on the part of donors that their funds are not desperately needed by the hospitals and are accepted with little clear sense of responsibility to the community from which they come. There is little purpose in donating funds to organizations that are essentially commercial, whatever their tax status. Many voices now call for stiffer conditions governing hospital exemptions from taxation,[18] and a clear separation between community and commercial institutions might well attract more philanthropy to community institutions in the long run. So might the establishment of a CHIB that would identify and manage the allocation of support to a cooperative, community-oriented stratum of institutions. While philanthropy could not in the near term meet all major capital funding requirements of a CHIB, CHIBs could and probably should encourage private donations.

DISTRIBUTION OF FUNDS

The CHIB should distribute its funds on the basis of its coverage, resources, and mission. Funds can be allocated for a variety of purposes:

- To maintain and upgrade physical facilities
- To provide adequate equipment and up-to-date technology
- To purchase or subsidize specific services
- To subsidize institutions
- To support community organizing, planning, and project development

Major Capital Support

Several options are available to the CHIB seeking to provide support for major construction and renovation projects. These include grants, loans, loan guarantees, and operating subsidies.

Grants. Grants are distributions of funds made without expectation of financial repayment. However, they are usually given for specified purposes to which the recipient institution is expected to adhere. In the Hill-Burton program, for example, grants were conditioned on detailed planning and adherence to architectural, equipment, and construction standards. Grants can be distributed in a single lump sum or in a series of lump-sum payments as construction proceeds. Hill-Burton adopted the latter approach. Grants can also be designed to retire indebtedness incurred by an institution to finance construction. Such grants might be disbursed monthly or in annual installments over the life of the bond or other obligation or be given in a lump-sum payment to retire all or a portion of the debt.

Installment payments would help a CHIB that is funded by a gradually increasing revenue diversion make major capital commitments more quickly. So would the use of its own (or the state's) credit to borrow to increase its pool of funds. In both cases, however, speed comes at the price of future financial flexibility because debt retirement will have first claim on future CHIB income. A CHIB is a fundamentally political organization organized to respond to a rapidly changing health care environment. Long-term commitments like these could extend the CHIB's financial commitments beyond the time when its current investment strategies make sense. Long-term financial commitments will also severely limit the ability of governors and legislatures to terminate or alter the CHIB in response to social changes. We would recommend that CHIBs avoid the temptation to borrow. They should limit their financial commitments to those they can meet with funds actually on hand.

Loans. Lending money does not create the same inflexibility that borrowing money does. If a CHIB lends money to institutions, primary responsibility for ownership and financing of the assets purchased with the funds could rest either with the borrowing institution or with the CHIB. If the institution assumed initial ownership, it would repay the CHIB's loan and the CHIB could assume ownership or acquire rights to intervene in its management if the institution defaulted. If the CHIB assumed initial ownership, the institution could "buy" the asset from the CHIB over time.

The CHIB's ability to lend funds depends, of course, on an expectation that the institution receiving the loan will be able to repay it from future operating revenues. If the recipient institution is an essential element in the community sector, it will know that the CHIB is committed to its continued survival even if it does not repay the loan, and may try less assiduously than a commercial-sector institution to maintain the financial strength necessary for repayment. Long-term loans also assume that the recipient ought to be in business for an extended period of time. As in the case of "installment grants" discussed previously,

CHIBs will need to evaluate loan situations with great care and incorporate strict monitoring and control provisions into the loans they make.

Loan guarantees. Loan guarantees are commitments to repay the borrowing obligations of institutions if they fail to make promised payments. Guarantees allow institutions to gain access to lenders who otherwise would not lend to them and to receive lower interest rates. The capital commitment required of the CHIB for a loan guarantee program is theoretically much lower than for a loan or grant program. But unless the CHIB makes a large number of such guarantees, it may still have to maintain a large reserve because a single default could consume all its resources. The best solution probably is to purchase reinsurance against the risk of default from an insurance company or from a loan guarantee pool established by a consortium of CHIBs. It is important to recognize that loan guarantees cannot substitute for grants when institutional financial capacity is simply too strained to retire major debt. Moreover, to qualify for reinsurance, a CHIB's guarantees would have to meet strict market tests. Thus, a CHIB program of loan guarantees would end up resembling existing public and private mortgage insurance programs. There seems little reason for a CHIB to spend its limited resources duplicating existing services.

Mortgage insurance. For the same reason, mortgage insurance itself probably does not offer an appropriate method of CHIB asset distribution. Insurance differs from a loan guarantee in that the institution pays a fee to the issuer in return for a repayment guarantee. A well-managed mortgage insurance operation will break even or make a profit, as do the federal government's HUD 242 program and several private mortgage insurance firms. Insurance rarely provides access to capital markets for institutions that otherwise would be denied—insurers refuse truly high-risk applicants. The most it does is lower the interest rates paid by institutions that already enjoy access. Moreover, insurance programs violate a basic principle of CHIB design because they do not allocate a fixed pool of funds. Given these problems, and in view of the fact that mortgage insurance is already available to hospitals and nursing homes through other suppliers, providing insurance seems not a useful activity for CHIBs to pursue.

Interest and operating cost subsidies. Interest and operating-cost subsidies can be used to provide access to private capital markets by improving an institution's ability to repay loans. For example, the state of New York sometimes modifies its cost reimbursement formulas for specific hospitals to allow them to qualify for federal mortgage insurance. Subsidies differ from grants, loans, and loan guarantees in at least one fundamental respect: rather than connecting the institution with sources of financial capital, they flow directly to the institution through its operating revenues and leave the institution to compete for access to private capital markets. In this sense, subsidies may be thought of as a form of prospective capital payment. Unlike standardized, formula-based capital payment, however, CHIB subsidies would be available only to selected institutions. Presumably CHIB subsidies would also be linked to specific capital investment proposals and to commitments to provide defined forms and levels of community service. Subsidies would permit a degree of ongoing influence over recipient attentiveness to these commitments. If a recipient institution did not honor the community service obligations it accepted when the subsidy contract was executed, the CHIB could terminate the subsidy. In such cases, the subsidy might be thought of as a series of renewable operating grants or purchase-of-service contracts.

The Hill-Burton experience demonstrates that planned capital payment programs should be able to provide operating as well as capital subsidies if they hope to choose investments with the greatest potential to improve health. Of course, in a state that maintains the general financial strength of its hospitals and other essential providers through a system of universal health insurance or a bad debt and free care pool, the need for operating or even physical capital subsidies might lessen or, conceivably, disappear. In fact, a system of universal health entitlement (or its financial equivalent), in which institutions could reasonably be expected to maintain their own financial stability on the basis of operating revenues, would create better incentives all around. The CHIB could concentrate on targetted capital and program investments and get out of the business of trying to decide whether the financial difficulties of an institution it subsidizes are due to indigent care, geographic isolation, or poor management. Payment for specific community-oriented services not covered by the entitlement system could be arranged on a contractual basis.

Purchase of Services

Closely related to interest and operating-cost subsidies designed to provide access to capital are grants and contracts for the provision of specific services. Both support the operating rather than the capital expenditures of institutions. Grants could be given to institutions to support their activities in general, much as an individual donates funds to the United Way or to a college. Alternatively, and probably preferably, funds could be allocated in response to proposals to meet a community need that the CHIB has identified, or for more routine services that the CHIB simply wants to buy on the community's behalf. The Hill-Burton program's success at prompting architectural and construction standards shows the value of clearly specifying the actions that the CHIB wants an institution to take in return for funds received.

Start-up Support and Technical Assistance

Finally, the CHIB could provide seed money, working capital, planning funds, and nonmonetary assistance to communities or institutions that desire to provide important services but lack the resources to compete with other applicants on equal terms. These forms of assistance might also afford the CHIB an opportunity to observe the competence and commitments of applicants that lack track records. Start-up assistance could be structured to require substantial commitments of sweat equity from such applicants so as to confirm further the seriousness of their commitment to community service. If technical and start-up assistance were provided to more groups than could ultimately be funded, it would help counteract the natural tendency to establish informal relationships and ties to organizations that may not, in the end, merit funding.

Summary of Fund Distribution Options

Obviously, CHIBs need not limit themselves to just one or even two of these distribution methods. However, it does appear that the most appropriate distribution methods for CHIBs to adopt are *grants, loans, operating subsidies, contracts for services* and *start-up support*. Each of these mechanisms can serve different sorts of applicants and require different behaviors from recipients, both before and after the award. Loans, for example, will attract only relatively financially healthy applicants and require them to manage themselves with a constant eye on the bottom line so as to avoid default. Grants will encourage institutions to exaggerate financial distress and possibly even to neglect cost management but will allow recipients to pay more attention to health needs in their day-to-day operations. Screens to exclude poorly managed institutions from receiving grants would have to be imposed. Some of the institutions that apply for grants also may have weak commitments to the CHIB's goals, unless the CHIB requires some form of substantial matching commitment on the applicant's part. Otherwise, grants may attract a mixed bag of applicants because they represent "free" money.

CHIBs that offer funds in two or more forms will have to avoid the temptation of overusing loans and loan guarantees in preference to grants simply because they appear to "go farther." Ultimately, this attitude can turn the CHIB into an organization guided by capital markets rather than by community needs, reduce its flexibility, and insulate it from desirable political control. Sophisticated management will be required to use all funding mechanisms effectively and to balance CHIB revenues, distributions, and strategic objectives over the long run.

A CHIB need not finance an entire project itself; it could ask all or some recipients to finance a portion. The institution's portion could be the same for all projects, or it could fluctuate in accordance with factors such as the CHIB's view of a project's desirability and the recipient's financing capacity. By having an adjustable rate of contribution, the CHIB would be able to provide full funding for financially distressed institutions and require better-endowed ones to pay a larger portion of a project's costs. It could further modify the institutional contribution based on a project's importance to the community. Similarly, the CHIB could vary the proportion of grant versus loan assistance that it offers. It could award grants to financially distressed institutions with high priority projects, and loans to other facilities at varying interest rates depending on the priority of the project and the financial strength of the borrower. Exhibit 4-1 illustrates how a CHIB might coordinate its form of fund distribution with project and institutional characteristics.[19]

Exhibit 4-1

Project Classifications with Loans and Grants

TYPE OF PROJECT	RECIPIENT CONTRIBUTION	LOAN/GRANT MIX
High-priority project in financially distressed institution	None	All grant, no loan
High-priority in well- or moderately well-endowed institution	Low	Possibly a small grant plus a low-interest loan
Medium-priority project in financially distressed institution	Low	Medium grant plus low-interest loan
Medium-priority project in well- or moderately well-endowed institution	High	No grant, medium- to high-interest loan
Low-priority project in any institution	Entire amount	Neither

PLANNING AND MANAGEMENT SYSTEMS

The CHIB envisioned by the mission, coverage, funding, and distribution mechanisms described above will be a large and complex organization. If it receives and redistributes funds within several sectors—say, general hospitals, long-term care, environmental health, medical education, and primary care—it will handle a large fund of money and manage a diverse portfolio of programs. If, as we recommend, it funds activities in these areas from a single resource pool that it controls, the CHIB will need to accomplish five distinct functions well.[20] It must:

- Budget funds from the general pool to broad categories of activity
- Identify priorities and strategies in each area of activity and create specific programmatic initiatives able to achieve them
- Evaluate requests for support, negotiate with applicants, and award funds
- Monitor institutional compliance with the terms of programmatic awards
- Evaluate the effectiveness of programs and periodically revise basic priorities and strategies.

In addition, of course, the CHIB must manage its funds carefully—a complex job when a variety of distributional mechanisms are used and multiyear projections and commitments are made. Finally, CHIBs must discharge all the other administrative responsibilities that attend the running of a sizable public or private organization.

Organizational design is a complex process that sometimes seems to depend as much on the strengths and preferences of an institution's leaders as it does on that institution's mission and environment. Organizations may need to be restructured simply to effect change, rather than because one structure is found to be consistently more efficient than another. We have seen the problems that attended federal attempts to specify detailed structures and management systems for local health planning organizations from afar, beginning with Hill-Burton. Nevertheless, details will matter as communities design CHIB planning and management systems. To indicate the design decisions that will have to be made and to spotlight some of the key details, we describe in the remainder of this chapter and in Chapter 5 a possible CHIB organizational design. This model CHIB exhibits several features that may be worth emulating. In this section, we discuss the organization of three essential CHIB activities: strategic budgeting, the awarding of funds, and program development.

We present first a brief overview of our entire model. Beginning at the top, we envision a board of directors or similar group that would exercise ultimate legal control over the CHIB's activities. (Exactly who should make up this board and how it would relate to government, political leaders, and interest groups are the subject of Chapter 5.) The board would hire and fire key CHIB executives. It would also establish the CHIB's annual and projected long-term strategic budget by authorizing the commitment of funds to major areas of support. By allocating these funds, the board would in effect divide its overall pool of resources into subpools committed to specified strategic objectives. In addition, within each subpool, the board could establish programmatic initiatives by issuing requests for proposals (RFPs). RFPs would describe activities that the board believes would be especially well suited to advancing the strategic objectives of subpools, thereby indicating the projects most likely to receive funds and helping potential applicants craft responsive proposals. Decisions to award funds would be made on the basis of a review of applications submitted by institutions; the board, itself, would approve all or most awards. There would be no requirement to award all the funds allocated to a given subpool or RFP within a given period, and the board would be free to shift funds among subpools and programs in each new strategic budget.

The bulk of the administrative structure of the CHIB would be organized around the subpools created by the board in its strategic budget. An operating division of the CHIB would be linked to each subpool. These divisions would evaluate and recommend action on applications for support, monitor the use of awarded funds, evaluate program effectiveness, and develop ideas for new or modified RFPs. Advisory committees would be created within each subpool to assist CHIB staff in all these functions. An executive director would coordinate and oversee the operating divisions.

In addition to the administrative apparatus devoted primarily to subpool management, there would be an independent staff responsible for preparing the strategic budget and for managing the aggressive process of public review and comment that would accompany each strategic budget cycle. As part of this job, this staff group would independently evaluate existing CHIB programs and scan the environment to identify changing needs and opportunities. The strategic budgeting and evaluation staff would report, not to the executive director, but to the chair of the board of directors—who would occupy a full-time, salaried position. Exhibit 4-2 shows an organization structured along these lines.

Exhibit 4-2
Proposed CHIB Organizational Structure

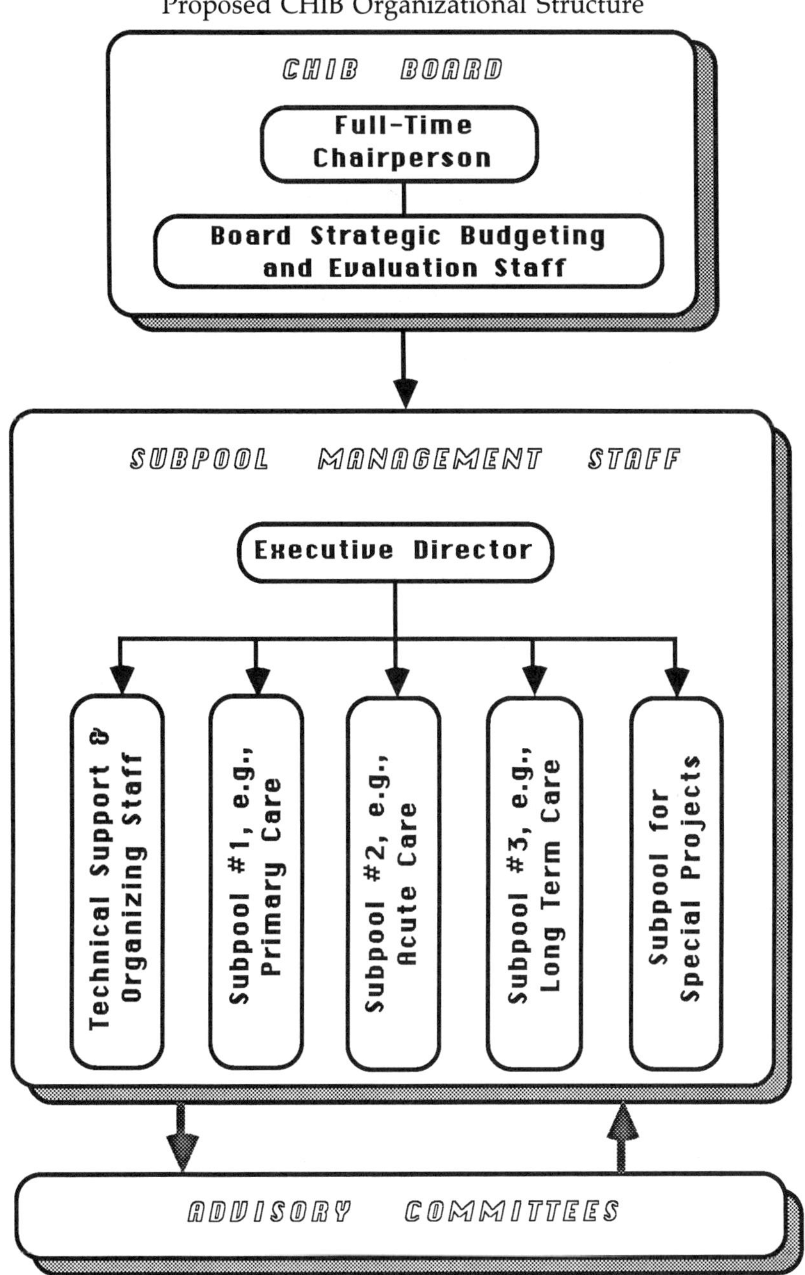

The Strategic Budgeting Process

The reader will note that nowhere in the preceding paragraphs does the word "plan" appear. This is intentional. Our hope is that little if any time will be spent on writing plans that resemble the health systems plans mandated by the National Health Planning and Resources Development Act or the state medical facilities plans required by Hill-Burton. Instead, we regard the annual strategic budgeting process as the CHIB's key planning activity, and we see the development and modification of this budget, together with the development of specific programmatic initiatives, as a flexible, opportunistic, steerable process that can, in a changing environment, invest CHIB funds where they will do the most good. We also see considerable merit in maintaining some separation between this strategic budgeting process, on the one hand, and the process of evaluating and choosing applicants for funds, on the other.

We envision strategic budgeting as primarily a top-down process to determine where funds ought to be spent to achieve the greatest public health benefit, with only partial regard to the present capacity of the health care system to absorb funds in any particular area. In other words, we are impressed with the power of money to stimulate over time the creation of institutions and programs to spend it, and we envision a strategic budgeting process that calls forth an institutional infrastructure that parallels actual health needs. In some cases, therefore, strategic budgeting would allocate funds to protected subpools without any immediate expectation that the allocated funds would be spent, and perhaps even before formal RFPs have been written to guide the spending. In other subpools, allocations might fall far short of the volume of funds that could be distributed if every qualified applicant received support. To further stimulate innovation, funds unexpended at the end of the year would remain within the subpool to which they originally were budgeted, unless reassigned by the board.

Through the strategic budgeting process, the board would annually or biennially dedicate its revenues to a series of strategic initiatives. Strategic budgeting on this model would require an ongoing ability to access and analyze epidemiologic data, and a thorough understanding both of the effectiveness of the CHIB's own programs and of programmatic alternatives worldwide. It would represent the key process by which a state or a community establishes its health infrastructure priorities for the noncompetitive sector. Therefore, the budgeting process should be a highly public exercise, involving the creation and circulation of a draft budget by the CHIB, consultation with many interests and points of view, and extensive public hearings. The process of review should attract more intense, more serious, and more helpful public participation than the health planning processes of the past because the allocation of real resources will be at stake. Representatives from various constituencies will be forced by the process to argue the relative merits of support for their own sector, since funds allocated to other sectors will be funds they do not receive. This should focus debate on precisely the "macro" strategic questions that a CHIB must face to act effectively, rather than on the "micro" institutional approval decisions that preoccupy CoN programs and other agencies that lack strategic budgeting authority.

By conducting a separate strategic budgeting process on the macro level, the CHIB should encourage more substantive and less cynical participation from its potential institutional clients. The stakes in the award process for an individual institution will not be obvious at the macro level. The precise effects of the board's programming and pool-creation decisions on particular projects or applicants will be hard for anyone to predict. That is part of the point of settling on priorities in advance. Even cynics will find it difficult to game the system at this stage. If, as a result, all energy is not consumed by calculations of particular advantage, then deliberation about community needs and strategies can be more rational and more substantive.

An important aspect of the strategic budgeting process for any CHIB will be the way it defines its subpools. A number of classifications can be imagined, such as the activity to be supported (new construction, renovation, support of services, or new project development) or the type of institution that will be funded (hospital, nursing home, or health center). A geographical division deserves to be considered, but we advocate a different grouping principle: *outcome*. The importance of judging the value of any investment or action by the outcome it causes is widely recognized. Outcomes give value to action. In principle, if potential uses of funds with a similar hoped-for outcome are grouped together in a single subpool, then decisions about how and to whom to allocate funds will turn on the relative ability of different alternatives to achieve the outcome. This is precisely the discussion one wants to encourage. Moreover, competition for funds would be open to a variety of kinds of institutions capable of producing the outcome of interest, so that grouping by outcome would encourage more innovation and a livelier debate over how best to achieve outcomes, while helping to prevent a single institutional constituency from capturing a given subpool.

Of course, any grouping by outcome (or other principle) will be an approximation, not an exact mapping. No two programs or institutions have exactly similar outcomes, and no truly useful program will have just one. Broad categories like primary care, acute care, medical education, and chronic care nevertheless share fundamental outcome orientations and are widely recognized by the general public. Primary care, for example, by most definitions encompasses screening, triage and referral, disease prevention, patient education, and reassurance. It can be provided through a variety of institutions, from community-controlled neighborhood health centers to hospital outpatient departments to HMOs to private physicians in solo practice. Primary care can also be linked to environmental health initiatives and to other community health programs.

Acute care concentrates on the cure or control of incapacitating or life-threatening illness: it employs its own characteristic institution (the general hospital), techniques, and professional relationships. Still, there are alternatives to hospitalization for many patients, and at least one of them–ambulatory surgery–has produced its own aggressive advocates and institutions. A wider spectrum of institutions compete to provide chronic care, ranging from decentralized home health care through intermittent respite care of various forms to care rendered by "total institutions" like nursing homes and skilled nursing facilities. Hospices and life-care communities represent important recent initiatives. However, the outcomes of all these chronic care institutions share a fundamental similarity, and every community needs a balance of services.

Sometimes there will be jurisdictional conflict about the proper subpool to which a program should be assigned. The process can be likened to the assignment of legislative bills to particular subcommittees. In addition, there may be special programs that a CHIB board wishes to single out for special attention and creative initiative; two obvious candidates are measures to treat and control AIDS and the provision of care to the uninsured. Or an application might challenge the settled convictions and interests of established pools. A "special projects" program or subpool would be a flexible budgeting device for the board, a way of signaling to the community of potential applicants that a special opportunity for funding exists, that special organizational efforts are hoped for, and that special selection criteria will be in force. Such a subpool might be created to support social HMOs and other vertically integrated managed care systems that produce a wider range of outcomes than the more focused subpools described in the preceding paragraphs.

There is, we think, another advantage in having a special projects program or subpool. By placing discretion in the hands of board members, it would in effect give the board additional operational control. If it found existing programs inadequate to a task, or the culture of existing operating divisions unsupportive, the board could give the job of exploring new options and possibilities to a special projects staff.

The Award Process

In contrast to the strategic budgeting activity, we regard the applicant selection activity as a bottom-up process that identifies who will receive support. As such, it will depend on a detailed knowledge of the applicant institutions, including their needs, aspirations, circumstances, and performance. As discussed in the Chapter 3 comparison of planned payment with CoN, the award process will work best if, for any given programmatic initiative, there exists a strictly limited pool of funds established in advance and if the CHIB uses this constraint to stimulate active negotiation with and among applicants.

The subpool managers and advisory groups responsible for making award recommendations to the board of directors should seek to identify the best combination of awards from among the available proposals. This implies an interactive process, because the first award in an area may well change the relative usefulness of related applications from neighboring institutions, and modification of the remaining applications might then be in order. For example, a decision to help finance conversion of hospital beds to a secure child psychiatric service might suggest that a competing application from a neighboring hospital be amended to provide nonsecure or outpatient services. It may even be that the most useful combination of awards is arrived at by denying funding to the application that is "best" individually, to fund a combination of awards that is best overall.

Obviously, decision making of this kind requires close staff involvement with the applicant institutions. The development of long-term relationships eventually would make objective strategic budgeting decisions impossible if there were no separation between the persons closely involved in recommending awards and the persons responsible for budgeting. This is one reason to build into the CHIB's organizational structure a clear separation between budgeting and award review. In addition, interactive, combinatorial selection is a group decision-making process, not primarily a paper-scoring exercise. To be effective, all the potential applications and institutions must be considered in one batch, and the review must be accomplished in stages to allow time for many options to be considered. (See in Appendix A the description of the Rochester HEP program's decision to fund a new mammography service for an example of how time, advisory committees, and interactive decision making can improve outcomes and identify important strategic issues.) This sort of review cannot realistically be undertaken by a board of directors with many other responsibilities and too little time to give extended consideration to any particular program. Anyone who has watched a busy regulatory commission in a large public meeting struggle to go beyond routine formulas and written staff analyses will appreciate the truth of this remark. Deliberations must occur and negotiations must be hammered out in relatively small groups whose members can spend all the time necessary to reach an informed conclusion. Active leadership at the staff level will be needed to make interactive selection work.

Extensive reliance on staff-guided decision making raises the problem that much of the decision-making process will be invisible to the board when it is asked to approve staff recommendations. By contrast, CoN decision making using explicit rules and standards may be cumbersome and misleading, but it creates a more transparent process and incorporates clearer guarantees of due process and fair treatment for applicants.[21] To help make the combinatorial selection process as fair and accountable as possible, we propose that advisory committees be created for each major award program, and that award deliberations be open to the public. Advisory committees would comprise—among others—representatives of the types of institution that are a program's potential beneficiaries. The committees would participate actively in award deliberations and would make an independent presentation to the board when it reviews staff recommendations for the approval of awards. Testimony from individual committee members and other observers would also be accepted, along with comments from institutional applicants.

Ultimately, however, extensive due process requirements are less necessary in a subsidy program of the kind we envision than in CoN because the CHIB will neither regulate institutions nor require the participation of institutions against their will. The CHIB's job is to spend money to achieve its mission as best it can. Institutions are not entitled to its funds, and it should have wide latitude to select its awardees as long as it does not discriminate by race, gender, or some other constitutionally or statutorily prohibited distinction.

Program Development

We envision that most if not all CHIB funds would be awarded on the basis of carefully thought-out programs, advertised by written requests for proposals, or RFPs, which the board would approve prior to publication. Each RFP would state as clearly as possible what the CHIB hopes to accomplish with the program in question, what sort of applications it seeks, and the criteria it expects to use to select the best combination of applications. Each RFP approval would include a specific "appropriation" for a pool of funds to finance the program; each appropriation would be deducted from the strategic budget allocation of a subpool.

To permit effective competitive decision making, competitions for a particular kind of support should be infrequent—every five years, for example—and a year or two of advance warning should be given to permit new organizations and previously unserved communities to develop competitive proposals. The board also should be able to carry over funds from year to year until an adequate pool of applications are in hand.

The RFP development process would occupy the middle ground between top-down strategic budgeting and bottom-up distribution of funds to institutions. The advisory groups and subpool staff that participate in the award process would also help develop proposals for new RFPs. Working in or close to a particular field, they should have a good sense of what existing institutions would like money to do and what it would be practical to ask institutions to undertake. They could also be expected to advocate more funding for their subpool and for the institutions with which they regularly work. We imagine an annual program development process through which the board would solicit program proposals from subpool managers and advisory groups, listen as these advocates argue the relative merits of their proposals, and eventually designate a limited set of proposals for development into formal RFPs.

In addition to this upward percolation of program ideas, the board will want to gain an independent, top-down perspective on programmatic needs and possibilities. An independent planning staff—the independence of which would be considerably enhanced if it were managed by a full-time board chairperson rather than by the executive director—should be established to perform this function. This staff could also manage the process of collecting and comparing program development proposals submitted from below.

ORGANIZATIONAL STRUCTURE

We summarize the basic organizational structure necessary to support the strategic budgeting, program development, and award distribution processes described previously in organizational chart form in Exhibit 4-2. To reiterate, we envision an organization of several operating divisions—one corresponding to each of its major subpool areas of support, plus possibly two or three other special divisions. Special divisions might be organized to provide financial analysis to the operating divisions, to monitor awardee compliance with the terms of CHIB support, and to handle special projects. Because the strategic budgeting process will, we recommend, organize subpools and their associated operating divisions on the basis of common outcomes, this structure is analogous to product-line management in private firms. Operating divisions would be given significant autonomy to achieve the outcomes delegated to them, and their performance would be measured in outcome terms.

In addition to the operating or product-line divisions, a special strategic planning group will be necessary to manage the board's deliberations, organize public hearings, evaluate CHIB programs, scan the environment, develop scenarios, and prepare macro-level strategic plans. All the divisions except the strategic planning group would report to an executive director, who would report to the board. The board would also establish advisory groups to assist in award selection and program development at the subpool or operating-division level. We discuss board composition and other issues related to governance and accountability in the next chapter.

NOTES

1. Gail R. Wilensky, "Solving Uncompensated Hospital Care," *Health Affairs* 3 (1984): 50–62.
2. One state, Pennsylvania, went so far as to issue an executive order for the creation of an allocation system in anticipation of congressional approval. Some observers expect Congress to impose a system of caps on tax-exempt health borrowing in the near future.
3. Strictly speaking, however, allocations from equipment pools are not planned but depend on a show of creditworthiness by the borrowing institution.
4. A colleague from the People's Republic of China, Dr. Lin Zihua, recently introduced me to a Chinese colloquialism that concisely captures the problem of a governmental agency trying to induce an action larger than its resources can command: "Lion's head, mouse's body."
5. There are strong arguments in favor of repealing CoN laws in states that establish CHIBs. To the extent that such state CoN programs also perform quality assurance functions—say, by imposing minimum staffing and equipment standards on new programs—these functions can be transferred to state licensure programs. To do so, states would have to issue licenses by service rather than merely by institution and, for services like open heart surgery and cardiac catheterization that depend on market entry limitations to preserve quality by maintaining program caseloads, states would have to add such systemwide considerations to the list of more traditional licensure standards. Better still, they could require periodic relicensure without a guarantee of grandfathering in order to cope with cardiac programs whose caseloads fall below safe levels sometime in the future.
6. Office of the Assistant Secretary for Planning and Evaluation, Department of Health and Human Services, *Hospital Capital Expenses: A Medicare Payment Strategy for the Future* (Washington, DC: U.S. Office of the Assistant Secretary, 1986), p. 30.

7. Gerard Anderson and Paul B. Ginsburg, "Prospective Capital Payments to Hospitals," *Health Affairs* 2 (Fall 1983): 52–63.
8. Office of the Assistant Secretary for Planning and Evaluation, *Hospital Capital Expenses*.
9. For a good critical synopsis of these estimates, see Donald R. Cohodes and Brian M. Kinkead, *Hospital Capital Formation in the 1980s* (Baltimore: Johns Hopkins University Press, 1984), pp. 27–34; Office of the Assistant Secretary for Planning and Evaluation, *Hospital Capital Expenses*, p. 126.
10. See, for example, Alain Enthoven, "Health Tax Policy Mismatch," *Health Affairs* 4 (Winter 1985): 5–14.
11. M. Susan Marquis, *Cost-Sharing and the Patient's Choice of Provider* (Santa Monica, CA: Rand Corporation, 1984).
12. For a good summary of the arguments against taxation of health insurance benefits, see Rashi Fein, *Medical Care, Medical Costs: The Search for a Health Insurance Policy* (Cambridge, MA: Harvard University Press, 1986), pp. 177–86.
13. Congress might wish to legislate some encouragement and guidance to HCFA in that agency's efforts to award such waivers.
14. Steven R. Estaugh, "Hospital Diversification and Financial Management," *Medical Care* 22 (1984): 704–23.
15. Jonathan Betz Brown, Russel Jacobson, and Lynn Jenkins, *A Survey of Hospital Corporate Restructuring*, Health Capital Project Working Paper #12 (Boston: School of Public Health, Harvard University, 1985).
16. The CHIB might be able to reduce aggregate debt service costs by consolidating systemwide debt. If so, specific arrangements would have to be made with each institution from which revenues are to be diverted to ensure that its debt retirement obligations can be met.
17. See Regina E. Herzlinger and William S. Krasker, "Who Profits from Nonprofits?" *Harvard Business Review* 87 (1987): 93–106 for a denunciation from the point of view of for-profit firms of the various tax advantages enjoyed by nominally nonprofit hospitals.
18. See, for example, Robert M. Sigmond, "Re-Examining the Role of the Community Hospital in a Competitive Environment," The Michael M. Davis Lecture, Center for Health Administration Studies, University of Chicago, 1985; and John K. Iglehart, "Health Policy versus Budget Cutting: A Conversation with Rep. Pete Stark," *Health Affairs* 5 (1986): 22–30.
19. The ideas in this paragraph and the accompanying exhibit are contributed by David W. Young, D.B.A., professor of accounting at Boston University School of Management and member of the Health Capital Project. They derive in part from Dr. Young's study of the Massachusetts Housing Finance Agency, which appears as Appendix B.
20. David W. Young developed an earlier version of this list.
21. Some CoN agencies, of course, are adept at using rules and due process requirements to force applicants to "deal." One thinks particularly of the New York program in this respect. Over the years, New York has managed to close hospitals without the regulatory power to do so by causing their creditors to demand immediate payment (the program published a list of hospitals that should close), and to force major Manhattan teaching hospitals to take small community hospitals in poor and minority neighborhoods under their wing as a condition of approving applications to rebuild. The main decision-making body in New York, the Hospital Review and Planning

Council, is large, busy, and accustomed to the delegation of considerable authority to Department of Health staff. The staff, in turn, is able, numerous, and sufficiently well paid to minimize turnover.

5.

Governance

Stephen R. Thomas

In this chapter we consider the governance of the community health infrastructure bank. For the sake of concreteness, we add more detail to the account of how a CHIB might be organized. In doing so, we make explicit the design criteria that we believe a CHIB ought to exhibit. Our question will be, how should the CHIB be related to state government in light of the patterns of politics that will surround the CHIB's decisions? We conclude with the suggestion that managed pluralism, as we call the upshot of our proposed design, can promote strategic planning and a fair recognition of multiple health objectives in various communities.

THE POLITICAL DESIGN TASK

Designing a CHIB is not a problem in optimization because there is no "objective function": we cannot specify in advance the exact outputs we want it to produce, the conclusions we want it to reach. The design problem is challenging because a CHIB will inevitably be an agenda-setting and problem-defining institution, not merely a problem-solving institution. It ought to have the capacity for deliberation, not just horse trading; strategic planning, not just project review.

A CHIB has public functions. It makes decisions on behalf of society, but so do many different types of governmental and quasi-governmental entities. Because the CHIB has public functions, both the outcomes it achieves and its means of achieving them should be subject to public scrutiny, if not necessarily to direct governmental control.[1] Later in the chapter, we suggest that the CHIB be organized within the executive branch of state government, but with less insulation from ordinary political control than other observers may want.

We care about the technical adequacy of a CHIB's decisions, but they can be evaluated only after we satisfy ourselves that a CHIB's pattern of decision making seems likely to define the health capital problem in a suitably comprehensive way and to encourage a broad canvass of community opinion and judgment. Capital decisions, as we have already said, shape a community's health care system—which is to say, they help shape the community itself.

Approaching health capital decisions from a political point of view means recognizing that our nation has, over time, made choices and established expectations that could have been otherwise. Our analysis of how a CHIB might be organized and how it might operate will contribute to an expanded political discussion that is both desirable and by now, we think, unavoidable.

At the same time, we know that no institutional reform could (or should) capture within one mechanism all the ways by which capital decisions in health care are made. Health policy is like energy policy or industrial policy or family policy: the adjectives by themselves do not tell us how wide the policy domains are or ought to be. Not only are the spillovers almost endless, but decision making is diffuse and decentralized. How much of the capital decision making (direct and indirect) in the health care delivery system should be drawn together into a more centralized system is itself a practical matter that states and communities must debate for themselves.[2] A nation invests not only in physical plant and equipment for health care (along with training and research) but also in the capacity to plan for its health care. Myriad capital-related policies contribute to this capacity to plan. How they are organized is an important subject of concern.

First we suggest some criteria that can be used to define improvements in that planning capacity. Then we review the kinds of arrangements that state legislators might consider in preparing, let us say, a bill to direct various funding sources into a capital pool. Such a proposal might be motivated by the prospect of a HCFA waiver allowing Medicare and Medicaid participation. Or, more modestly, a legislature might be looking for an orderly way to direct general revenues or federal grants in support of the capital requirements and programs of deserving hospitals.

CRITERIA

On what basis should HCFA or a state legislature judge the adequacy of a state's proposed CHIB structure? What range of probable outcomes is acceptable? What features of the proposed process of decision making itself should Congress and HCFA care about? What kind of politics ought to be encouraged, and how?

Answering such questions, however tentatively, requires care and sophistication in order to avoid a mechanistic, Tinkertoy theory of government. These questions of policy design link substance and political process; legislators and executive agencies always address them in practical circumstances and in the course of legislative debate. They are part of the "middle game" of politics, where high-minded objectives may or may not be connected with effective measures.[3] To those in the business of keeping close track of proposals affecting them, the stakes will be plain: "Organization," a political scientist once observed, "is the mobilization of bias in preparation for action."[4] Organizational arrangements are never neutral in their effects, though their effects are often unintended or unforeseen. Governmental policies and their implementation do more than just respond to political preferences; governmental programs create new patterns of politics, indeed new constituencies.[5]

We mention the main characteristics that the CHIB ought to exhibit to clarify the design issues that would arise in a legislative debate about such a scheme. Specifying them also helps indicate what the politics would be like.

Accountability

Accountability can refer to several different issues. Who will take political responsibility for the decisions? How can the issues be framed so that parties besides providers and other, directly affected professionals will understand what is at stake? How can the articulation of a broad range of views be assured? Accountability refers to control, especially to official and formal control. One can tell to whom one is accountable—to a bureaucratic superior, a political head, a constituency.

Substantive Competence

We have already mentioned the analytic work that the CHIB will oversee and use (see also Appendix B). The board, and most especially the executive director, will ultimately be responsible for developing the necessary technical capacity and professional ambience. Applicants for CHIB support together with CHIB's various program-specific advisory groups would have an interest in the quality of the CHIB's staff work.

Representation

The administrative arrangements we choose will inevitably affect the relative influence of various interested parties. We can try to fix existing imbalances in influence, and thereby reshape outcomes, by tinkering with where decision-making bodies are located and how they are organized. But our proposal to make the CHIB a regular part of state government is a decision to work with the existing forms of political representation, rather than construct new representative bodies (like the much-maligned HSAs).[6] We will want the CHIB to shape the way interests get represented in the allocation process. We think that advisory committees, appointed by the CHIB board and each associated with one of several programs or subpools, will help focus the attention of existing constituencies on the CHIB's business. Still, we should not assume that only "interest groups" deserve representation. The CHIB board and the advisory bodies should be prepared to hear opinions relating to larger communities, and they will need professional recommendations and evaluations as well.

Board members, in this scheme, would not be group representatives in any formal way, but they will inevitably have strong ties to one or another health constituency; that is part of their value, after all, to the governor's administration. But we want the board to take a broad view. It would fund subpools and authorize programmatic initiatives, then review program staff recommendations regarding specific awards of funds.

Each subpool would have an advisory committee, appointed by the CHIP board. We think the board would be well advised to name members to each committee who represent the groups most affected by, or most knowledgeable about, that program's actions.

Participation

The CHIB will provide an additional focus for existing forms of political participation: elections, administrative process (including public hearings), legislative oversight, and opportunities to influence the publicity surrounding the CHIB's actions. Participants in the process will include organized provider groups (hospitals, physicians, other medical care providers), payers (including Medicaid), various consumer and advocacy groups, interested citizens, and local governmental officials.

We take public participation seriously because we think public input can, at least over time, help raise the quality of CHIB decisions by subjecting professional opinion to probing and challenging questions and by providing better information about community views and feelings. There is a constant pressure toward "imbalanced political markets."[7] Increased opportunities for participation in specialized public business may also, over time, contribute to a more informed, competent, and responsible citizenry.[8] Unlike some of the more ambitious historic reforms, ours would stress not the machinery of participation but the incentives to participate, lest the machinery create unintended biases and new disappointments.

Occasions for public input exist at distinct levels of decision making. We characterize them as follows:

- –Legislative decisions: the CHIB design, state appropriations if any
- –Major strategic decisions about programs: creation of subpools and RFPs for programs within subpools, annual allocations of CHIB program funds to the subpools, program staffing levels, rule making to govern the determination of awards to institutions
- –Evaluation of proposals: staff rankings or recommendations (subject to public hearing), public meetings of advisory committees (advisory committee comments accompany staff report to CHIB board)

At each stage, we want there to be opportunities not only for constructive political negotiation but also for a more exploratory, iterative process of mutual clarification of positions and joint learning.

Deliberative Capacity

The capacity we have in mind here is desirable in executive-branch committees and boards no less than in legislatures. We said earlier that the CHIB would set agendas and define problems. We also want the CHIB to plan strategically, implement plans effectively, and maintain public confidence. If the CHIB succeeds in that, it may add to public understanding of the hard choices in health care, as well as to its own knowledge of how to proceed. Strategy, effective implementation, and political legitimacy go together. They are linked by the capacity of the agency to explore options candidly, sometimes identifying new possibilities as it goes, and to explain alternatives clearly. This means that the

CHIB would not just record deals struck in the great game of American pluralism, but would at least sometimes succeed in raising the level of play.

By strategy, we mean the articulation of objectives in light of resources and circumstances. Strategy is thought in the service of prior goals and future action. It is rhetoric for the new age of large-scale organization. To think strategically is to craft goals in light of circumstances and to change what can be changed, the better to pursue the goals. Strategic planning is planning whose purpose is not to write a plan but to makes real choices—to adjust one's own organization so as to be in a position to act more effectively.

Strategy is hardly automatic in any kind of organization, even one in which there is a single "bottom line" and where competitive market forces are unmistakable. There can be such a thing as corporate strategy because there is such a thing as management, but managers may or may not act strategically. In the public sector, strategy is especially problematic because: (1) financing typically comes from legislative action for specified purposes and often for specific constituencies and comes accompanied by multiple constraints on agency action; (2) programs almost always have multiple objectives, and their accomplishment is usually hard to measure—a big part of strategy is therefore problem definition (there is not even the luxury of an all-purpose rule like "maximize shareholders' equity"); and (3) in an environment of (deliberately) fragmented power, managers may have more influence with the coalitions that sustain them than over their own personnel. In effect, strategy often precedes management and is much less amenable to change than the word implies.

A STATE PERSPECTIVE

We favor appointment of the CHIB board by the governor, with the advice and consent of the state senate, for terms of office coinciding with the governor's own and renewable at the governor's pleasure. The board would function as part of a broad multipurpose secretariat or within the purview of a cabinet council. The idea is to serve the governor's political priorities by providing some general management input, some locus for integrative staff work on health policy within the state.

The state legislature is also a source of political control. The CHIB would require an enabling statute and legislative support for a Medicare waiver, for example, and the state legislature would be heavily involved in providing other sources of financing for the CHIB.

Will the legislature interfere by overriding decisions made by the CHIB? Losers would no doubt make appeals to the legislature, as has happened in the CoN process. But we believe that the structure we propose would give the CHIB political clout to resist legislative interference on behalf of disappointed applicants. While in unusual circumstances a legislature might appropriate new funds for a particular facility or community program, we think that legislators would normally recognize the advantages of letting the CHIB make these tough decisions.

Of course, a legislature might act punitively: for example, holding up appointments or cutting the CHIB budget as a way of sending the governor a message. But again, while we cannot eliminate the possibility, the legislature is more likely, we think, to want the CHIB to take the heat than to want to second-guess its occasionally unpopular decisions.

Why do we choose to make the CHIB an entity of state government? One answer is that, to a greater degree than any alternative, the states have the ability to take on this job. They are familiar, subnational political entities, commanding legitimacy and political loyalty. Their boundaries are arbitrary, true, but like proverbial good taxes, they are also old. State governments seek to advance a wide variety of public purposes and can (often, though not always) focus attention on the choices that must be made among competing public investment objectives. As established political communities, the states can mobilize consent more effectively than substate entities created for a special purpose.[9]

The boundaries of a state are settled, and they are arbitrary: only by accident will they satisfy the strictures of regional finance or the economies of scale afforded by some particular technology. In addition, there may be significant political cleavages within a state that must be recognized: New York, California, and Illinois have especially big internal cultural and political variations. Arguments can be made on both technical and political grounds for creating substate regional CHIBs. We assume that such arguments will be made at the state level, and we assume that technical criteria will be regularly sacrificed to political expediency. We leave those matters to the states and would not try to constrain their decisions at the federal level. Substate CHIBs would remain accountable to state government, each one presumably with its own strategic budgeting and project review processes.

State government can improve the way decisions are made regarding capital allocations for health care facilities by helping to correct the effects of other policies. Whether they allocate their own funds or organize mechanisms for evaluating projects funded by federal capital funds, they can focus the debate on distributional issues and on the trade-offs with other worthy objects of public expenditure. Moreover, states would have a fiscal stake in the decisions of the "banks," because of Medicaid. Health systems agencies (and comparable planning entities in other program areas) do not have these characteristics.[10] In "strong governor" states, it may also be possible to use a CHIB to pull together programs that can trip each other up (or interfere with the CHIB) and that deserve coordination.

We choose states not for legalistic or ideological reasons but on pragmatic grounds. In light of national capital markets and multistate "corporate" medicine, however, state responsibility for strategic planning in health care must be squared with legitimate national objectives. Cost containment, limiting the liability of the federal government in financing health insurance (and medical research), is such an objective, but it is obviously not the only one. Everyone's access to some minimal amount of health care is a widely acknowledged norm, whatever the conceptual ambiguities and shortfalls in practice, and minimal "amount" includes the specification of both the services or procedures to which people have a right and their quality. States will vary in the health services available within their borders; practice patterns among physicians are unlikely to become perfectly uniform; individuals will continue to be able to afford differential kinds and amounts of medical care. We see no realistic way to eliminate these differences altogether. State performance in health planning ought not to be judged in accordance with objectives that the nation either does not know how to define or has not chosen to set for itself. In short, a state's political culture must, for the sake of effective implementation, be respected. By the same token, under existing Medicare policies the federal government will have to set minimum criteria for participation in a waiver.

In the next section we consider the main choices available to a state, and we say more about the potential value of planning by general government, compared to the alternatives. Cooperation among health care institutions does not require government, and government does not necessarily stifle voluntary community efforts to organize and finance human services of various kinds. This much is plain from the Rochester area example detailed in Appendix A. But it is also true that governmental inducements are sometimes required to break logjams and to lend authority to unwelcome tasks like reducing a region's acute bed capacity. Public authority that only government can provide can also push the horizons of debate outward and prevent existing interests from controlling the health agenda.

OPTIONS

Any legislative or wider political debate about how to structure the operations of a CHIB is about machinery and politics, about how organization affects relative advantage and foreseeable outcomes. While there are matters of general principle to review, we must also pay attention to how formal arrangements affect the incentives of the players in the health care system. Debate about principles seems more high-minded, and it may sometimes be a screen for the bloodier business of goring oxen.

Kaufman's classic discussion of the organization of state government distinguishes three values pursued in various historic periods, each dominating opinion and practice in turn: representativeness, neutral competence, and executive leadership. Each principle has a good argument, and "the shift from one to another generally appears to have occurred as a consequence of the difficulties encountered in the period preceding the change."[11]

We think of an appropriate CHIB design as giving each of these principles its due. Health planning can aim for too much representativeness and wind up with too little. Neutral competence—legal and administrative autonomy for expert bodies—has often led to fragmentation, intellectual incoherence, and capture by directly affected groups. The CHIB we propose shows the dominance of the principle of executive leadership, allowing if not assuring political responsibility and explicit trade-offs among public objectives at the state level.

Legislatures have sometimes chosen to insulate specific regulatory or resource allocation functions from the normal vagaries of politics. The underlying idea is that the integrity of the process and the quality of the decisions need to be protected from shortsighted amateurs, narrow-minded partisans, and the pressures of political patronage. Classic ways of accomplishing this insulation include independent commissions, authorities, and special districts. Is any of these structures appropriate for the CHIB?

In some respects, authorities and commissions, special-purpose districts and independent boards, are of a piece in state and local government. They all divide power into functionally and often geographically distinct parts, leaving less direct political leverage in the hands of the elected officials responsible for running general government. That, of course, was historically part of the intention. Businesslike government was government taken out of the hands of the ethnic machines. "Good government" is also less-visible government and, often, government offering new kinds of sinecure.

Regulatory Commissions

In their classical embodiments, independent regulatory commissions exercise powers that are quasi-legislative and quasi-judicial. Having both types of power distinguishes commissions from ordinary executive agencies, even other regulatory agencies. Their legislative function is typically in accordance with an especially broad delegation of authority from a legislature. The decisions entrusted to commissions, moreover, arguably affect rights – property rights – in an especially sensitive way. The legislative mandates of the classic commissions have therefore interpreted due process to require commissions to be independent of political control and to act like courts. For this reason, commissioners do not serve at the pleasure of the executive but for fixed, and normally staggered, terms. Confirmation is by the legislature, sometimes by extraordinary majorities. A chief executive can exercise control, but less directly and quickly than over his executive departments, through the budgetary and appointment processes. But there are limits to how much a commission's budget can be strangled before the courts intervene to protect the legislatively mandated independence of the commission.[12]

Other Commissions

At the state level, commissions are organized in a variety of ways for a variety of purposes. The name sometimes betokens some special feature that sets the agency apart from the run-of-the-mill executive department, giving its decisions some degree of legal independence from normal political control. Insurance rates and Medicaid reimbursement rates are often set through legally protected procedures. In Massachusetts, the Metropolitan District Commission – responsible for the parks and recreational facilities (and until recently the water and sewer services) in the Boston metropolitan area – is a multipurpose special district. Its creation allowed member towns to keep the rates they were charged low; nonmember towns could protect their interests through legislative control of bonding authority.[13]

We do not find any good reason for CHIBs to be organized as commissions if that entails being agencies apart, with legally protected autonomy within state government. A commission CHIB would, we fear, wind up embodying the pretense, the often well-intentioned fantasy, that in matters of health care, expert authority should be given an extrapolitical preserve from which to accomplish the public good.

Health is widely regarded as special, requiring that deference be accorded the authority and expertise of the medical profession. Sometimes, as in the New York Hospital Review and Planning Council, memberships are by law reserved for physicians or other professionals. That council performs a regulatory function under the state of New York's CoN and licensure programs, and the same argument will no doubt be heard on behalf of a commission acting as a CHIB.[14] However, health capital planning should not be defined as a matter of professional medical judgment.

This model for a state commission puts physicians and other health professionals together with other interested parties, including representatives of "the public" or "consumers." Health planning has a tradition of special, areawide, representative bodies.[15] But some would argue for a further modification. "Commission" here would refer not only to the special qualifications for appointment, perhaps requiring nominations from specified groups, but also to fiscal independence from the rest of the executive branch. If such a commission made its annual budget requests and other recommendations directly to the legislature, bypassing the normal executive channels of review, it would ill-suit a CHIB, which, we argue, should not be isolated from the normal deliberative and administrative processes of general government. (As for federal funds, such a commission would exercise authority, under a waiver, to allocate the state's allotment of pooled funds.)

Authorities

This form of public agency is more standardized than the commission. To the autonomy of the appointment process (and therefore freedom from ordinary control), an authority adds financial autonomy: the power to finance projects through its own bonding authority. In a nation whose basic political institutions have many other remarkably archaic features, the rediscovery and development of the authority in the twentieth century is an example of genuinely inventive refurbishing. Spawned in the spirit of reform, authorities have sought not so much to improve government as to avoid it.

Robert Moses, the builder of New York City, was the chief architect of the public authority in its native guise. Like the man himself, his biographer Robert Caro writes, public authorities have been

> outside and above politics [Moses said]. Their decisions are made solely on the basis of the public welfare, he said. They have all the best features of private enterprise. They are businesslike—prudent, efficient, economical. And they are more. They are the very epitome of prudence, efficiency, economy. And they have another advantage over conventional governmental institutions as well. Since they finance their projects through the sale of revenue bonds to private investors, they therefore build these projects without using any public funds. Projects built by authorities, he said, cost the taxpayers nothing.
>
> These statements were believed implicitly for almost forty years by the public to which they were made. And this is not surprising. For Robert Moses repeated his contentions a thousand times and for four decades they were repeated, amplified and embellished by a press that believed them, too.[16]

Moses found a way to alter the statutory underpinnings of authorities so as to create a self-renewing financial base for vast personal political influence. Thanks to Robert Caro, Moses will forever be associated with the abuse of this financial and legal entity.

But authorities were also encouraged by the New Deal. The Tennessee Valley Authority is the most notable example. The Reconstruction Finance Corporation and the Public Works Administration made federal grants available to self-liquidating projects, thus encouraging fiscally troubled municipalities to organize authorities to undertake public works. Whether the money came from the federal government or from revenue bonds, the main inducement for the creation of authorities was financial independence from government's normal fiscal policies and problems.[17]

An authority provides access to the debt market for a public purpose that regular government either cannot or will not support from general revenues. An authority is the reply of "neutral competence" to politics and taxes. Similar independence will sometimes be harnessed to provide a conduit for the credit of others at below-market rates of interest. For example, the Massachusetts Housing Finance Agency (MHFA, patterned after New York's Housing Finance Authority) makes mortgage and construction loans to developers for new or rehabilitated housing. Major financial support for the agency's programs comes from the sale of tax-exempt revenue bonds, and the agency also dispenses federal and state housing program money. The MHFA imposes various standards and requirements (see Appendix B), including tenant mix, but the financing is attractive. And, Martha W. Weinberg explains, "although the developer's profits from the project are limited by MHFA, this limitation does not take into account the profits from which developers make the greatest amount of money, which come from their sale of limited partnerships in the project to individuals as tax shelters."[18]

The MHFA's 7-member board includes ex officio the cabinet-level heads of the state's Departments of Community Affairs and Corporations & Taxation. The governor appoints the other 5 members to seven-year terms. By law, one member must have mortgage banking experience, one must come from architecture or city and regional planning, and one from real estate. The governor also appoints a 15-member advisory committee. The executive director and the staff are not subject to civil service and serve at the pleasure of the board.[19]

Unlike a CHIB, the Housing Finance Agency does not operate under a cap. The MHFA tries to expand a good, not ration it and redistribute it. And, while a CHIB might be financed in part through bonding, that would limit its effect. The CHIB is aimed at making a bigger dent in existing financial and political behavior. The MHFA's success, Weinberg notes,

> hinges on whether it can sell bonds and provide capital for housing as well as private sector institutions can. . . . The social purpose of providing good housing often rides in on the back of satisfying the private market. For example, the MHFA staff has always been able to argue that without high-quality construction and without amenities such as swimming pools and recreation centers, their developments would not be rented by those who pay market rents.
>
> The market appeals to the self-serving interests of everyone involved. Developers make profits. Individual investors can find highly satisfactory tax shelters. Bondholders receive tax-free interest. The housing stock is increased, with all levels of income groups mixed in high-quality housing.[20]

We have doubts that this is a promising model of CHIB governance. The MHFA has legal and political autonomy of the kind we think is undesirable for the CHIB. But its operations suggest a scoring system that the CHIB staff and board might find suitable for evaluating projects within the limits of a particular RFP.[21] (See Appendix B for more on the MHFA and its scoring system.)

Clearly, a state's choice of an authority to exercise at least some of the functions of a CHIB would emphasize off-budget financing of capital subsidies.[22] Once that decision was made, other advantages of independence from ordinary political control would seem to follow—for example, a favorable bond rating based on the businesslike performance of the authority in evaluating projects. Authorities have personnel systems independent of regular civil service (usually implying higher salaries), preferable from a managerial point of view. The kind of professionalism that impresses financial markets is easier to achieve where an authority's board is remote from political control. That is one of the main purposes of authorities, to resist at least the more crass and democratic forms of politics. In doing so, they develop their own constituencies of beneficiaries, both consumers and creditors. And they put the state financially at risk, even in the absence of regular political accountability.[23]

When authorities proliferate, as they have in recent years, these special bodies—created to operate under their own statutes, and to serve particular "public purposes"—erode the power of general-purpose government.

> While each authority may have been justified on its own merits, the combined effect of these efforts has been to place the state in a precarious situation in which many of its most critical functions are performed by autonomous, non-elected governmental units. Just as no fiscally prudent individual would hand over his/her resources to a financial "expert" without demanding a detailed accounting of that expert's stewardship, so too, the Commonwealth should require a complete statement of how its resources are being used. Do we continue to entrust the Commonwealth's resources to autonomous authorities, or do we begin to take control of our finances and their allocation in a responsible and accountable fashion?[24]

There are two main issues of concern here. One is a regular accounting of activities to the executive and legislative departments. In Massachusetts (and we presume in other states), there is no such regular accounting; the boards are in charge, responsive to the authorities' constituencies and (at least formally) to the governor who appoints or reappoints. But even if there were regular reports, the main issue would persist. Off-budget financing (whether by revenue bonds or by trust funds, as in the federal highway and Medicare programs) does not permit policy trade-offs to be made at the margin. Its purpose is not to allow these trade-offs.

We are skeptical, to say the least, of the relevance to CHIB objectives of the nonpolitical independence, insulated expertise, and fiscal autonomy that lies behind enthusiasm for authorities. Sometimes they provide high-quality performance, sometimes not, and even professional performance may sacrifice legitimate public objectives that the CHIB, unlike an authority, is meant to pursue.

Special Districts

An authority can be thought of as one kind of special district, but there are differences. Districts–for example, school districts–have political and often some financial independence of other local government, and their boundaries may or may not match those of a single city or town. Their purpose is to perform some function or well-defined set of interrelated functions more efficiently and effectively than local general government. A district's governing officials may be appointed by local or state authority, or they may be elected as they often are in New England.[25] They collect tax money, and when they go to the debt markets, they do it on the strength of their taxing authority.

Special districts subdivide and disperse local power in the name of efficiency. They are based on a picture of government as a bundle of functions and services that can be organized separately; the beneficiaries of each service or function pay for it while at the same time operations, reaching across political boundaries, can exhibit economies of scale.

There are two principal effects of government by special district and by other functionally specific devices. One is that governmental decisions are visible mainly to those who benefit directly or lose directly, and who thus have an incentive to concentrate their fire.[26] Local economic and real estate interests gain at the expense of broader conceptions of the public interest. The other is that general government is likely to be less effective as functions and resources are partitioned off in the name of "good government." Power that is formally divided is power less likely to be exercised. That, of course, is the point of dividing it in the first place. Political "machines" and local creative entrepreneurship are two ways of putting power back together again, each having its own effects on the "public interest."[27]

THE CHIB AND MANAGED PLURALISM

These structural options are likely to appear as precedents in any legislative debate about a proposal like ours. These precedents appear, on reflection, to be mostly false trails. But formal structure is only part of our problem. We are interested in how structures affect the behavior of players in the process. We have, as Chapter 2 made clear, two principal worries: capture and irresponsibility. Keeping the foxes out of the chicken coop is important, but the chickens themselves will not necessarily remember the overall objective of their care and feeding. Autonomy must be squared with responsible political control.

There are, as usual, trade-offs to be made. On balance, the general government approach seems preferable. There are, of course, no guarantees. We can expect that unsuccessful applicants for CHIB-controlled funds will find that the design of planned payment is off, or that its procedures have been egregiously ignored. Some cynical observers of state government, perhaps emboldened by current fashions in free-market libertarianism, will reject the notion that a public agency can contribute anything useful to a health care system just now shaking off the effects of past regulatory blundering.

There can be some safeguards against capture and irresponsibility. Our CHIB proposal tries to include them in its overall design. We want CHIB operations to induce a broad range of interested parties to come forward. We can think of this pattern of administrative politics as "managed pluralism."

Managed pluralism refers to arrangements within the CHIB that are intended (1) to prevent capture by some (narrow) beneficiaries at the expense of others, and (2) to promote at the same time its own broad-gauged ability to deliberate wisely and act strategically. These objectives are, we think, in keeping with the historic arguments for political pluralism. Pluralism has aimed at containing the ambitions of any single group (government by coalition and plurality). And pluralism has sought to ensure that somewhere in the hurly-burly of pressure group politics there will be the capacity for deliberation; indeed, theory recognizes that multiplying and diversifying interests help make deliberation possible.[28]

The most important decision the CHIB board makes is to define the several programs that are funded in a given year by the several subpools also created by the board (see Exhibit 5-1). Program definitions are statements of objectives; they are devices for internal communication with

Exhibit 5-1
Proposed CHIB Governance Relationships

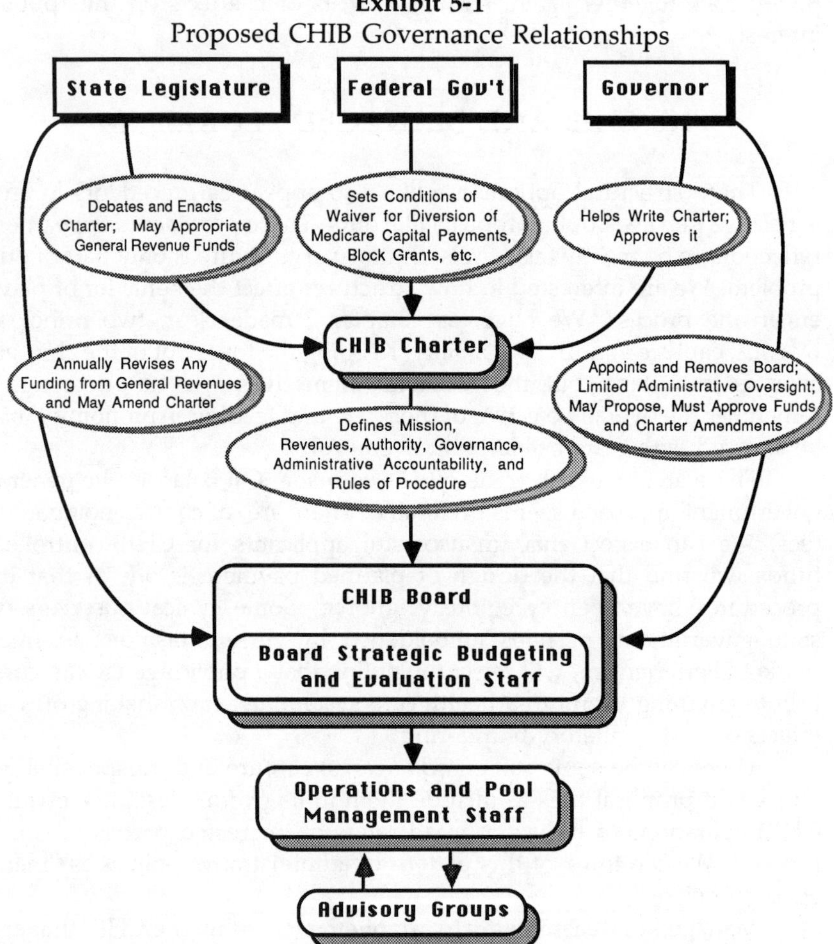

staff and advisory committees; and they are in effect requests for proposal from the CHIB's various constituencies. We think of these programs or subpools as being organized around particular kinds of care; they refer to output, not to type of institution (though they may map closely with type of applicant). For the sake of concreteness, we hypothesized several examples in Chapter 4, including acute care, long-term care, primary care, and prevention or promotion.

The board would have final approval of the staff's assignments of RFPs to specific pools. Given the existence of a cap on available funds for all projects, this budgetary decision is the crucial expression of the CHIB's priorities in a given period. It is analogous to the congressional budget process—the budget resolution for health capital expenditure, as it were.[29] The distribution to subpools will occur, to be sure, in anticipation of competition at the program level and in that context. (That is as it should be: the board's decisions creating and funding the subpools are strategic, but they are neither abstract nor apolitical.) Still, the precise effects of the board's programming and pool-creation decisions on particular projects or applicants will be hard for anyone to predict, although decisions about the more high-sounding matters will eventually affect specific players. That is the point of settling on priorities in advance. The debate should reflect this indeterminacy. Even cynics will find it difficult to game the system at this stage.

While the game will be zero sum soon enough, there are several games possible and some variations in the rules. In effect, the players have their own pregame, strategic choices to make, and they involve themselves in the community in order to make them. If on these strategic planning occasions, all energy is not consumed by calculations of particular advantage, then it is possible that genuine community feeling, a scarce commodity no doubt, can come to the fore and, in time, become less scarce.

Managed pluralism continues at the level of subpools and advisory committees. A program created by the CHIB board defines eligibility for would-be applicants. Strategy brings forward a constituency by targeting benefits. Each of the programs has an advisory committee, appointed by the board (after the consultations that one would expect, but according to no formalized procedure). Members of these committees serve for overlapping terms (of perhaps three years), but can be replaced at any time by a majority of the board. We would expect most members to come from the parts of the health care community most directly affected by specific programs, but we do not favor specifying in the CHIB charter their professional qualifications or organizational affiliations.[30]

Whether or not their memberships are formally defined by law, the program-specific advisory committees will have people from different organizations and various professions. The CHIB and its various constituencies need—politically as well as intellectually—diverse perspectives, and appointing experts who do not agree will be easier for the governor than appointing similarly divided amateurs. These appointees will, we hope, become loci for discussion and bargaining about the relative merits of specific types of project.

Proposals might be quite straightforward: facility modernization, new medical equipment, start-up support for new programming. After the manner of foundations, the CHIB might use eligibility to encourage new organizational forms (managed care innovations, for example) or cooperation among existing providers. The CHIB might, for example, seek to induce existing hospitals in a given locale to imitate the Rochester Area Hospitals' Corporation–in effect creating local pools, each with its own allocation mechanism for the local members.

The CHIB might want to use funds not only for planning grants to get things going in new directions, but also to support the participation of underrepresented groups in a particular area. We applaud this objective, although we recognize that particular states must decide for themselves whether to try to alter the configuration of interests in health care through such means. A state's CHIB statute might be permissive with respect to community organizing, allowing the CHIB itself discretion to use funds in this reformist fashion.

A final word. Our initial review of capital policy suggested how easy it is for policies to work at cross purposes. Existing policy was not designed from a single point of view or for a unified set of objectives, and it was not built in a day. In this context, our proposal has wide-ranging implications, but it tries to recognize the diversity and dynamism of the existing health care system.

Thus, the CHIB model we propose would complement and stimulate an emerging pattern of managed care in the United States. It is intended to give government a modest institutional lever to use in shaping (not determining) that system and correcting its shortcomings: to do what markets cannot do and to pursue objectives that we do not expect of competition. The public attitudes we would foster require new institutional forms to nurture them: not health planning old style, not regulation, not wide-eyed regionalism, but rekindled community involvement and a vital sense of governmental purpose.

NOTES

1. The CHIB's decisions are on behalf of society in two senses. First, in helping to shape the community's health care system, the CHIB contributes to a community's expectations regarding health–to the prevailing conception of health as a "socially defined good." See Michael Walzer, *Spheres of Justice* (New York: Basic Books, 1983); also Dan E. Beauchamp, "What Is Public about Public Health?" *Health Affairs* 2 (Winter 1983): 76–87. Second, the CHIB distributes capital across competing projects, and its decisions express the community's values about worthwhile goals.
2. In his Godkin lectures at Harvard, Senator Daniel Patrick Moynihan recently noted that "family policy is no one's business at present. . . . [T]he policy is . . . implicit and the only question is whether it is to be avowed. It was implicit in the tax code, in the budget, in child-support practices. But being no one's business, for the longest time no one noticed." Cited by Dennis Wrong in his review of Moynihan's *Family and Nation* (New York: Harcourt Brace Jovanovich, 1986) in *The New Republic* (March 17, 1986): 32. But once policy is explicit and avowed, it is hard to know where to stop the avowals: everything

government does affects the family. The question of boundaries cannot be answered except provisionally and pragmatically.

3. Laurence E. Lynn, Jr., *Managing the Public's Business: The Job of the Government Executive* (New York: Basic Books, 1981).
4. E.E. Schattschneider, *The Semi-Sovereign People: A Realist's View of Democracy in America* (New York: Holt, Rinehart & Winston, 1960), p. 30. Bruce Vladeck makes the same point in a fine paper on health planning. "In government," Vladeck writes, "anatomy is destiny." "Interest-Group Representation and the HSAs: Health Planning and Political Theory," *American Journal of Public Health* 67 (January 1977): 23.
5. For a short discussion that includes examples from health policy, see Lawrence Brown, *New Policies, New Politics: Government's Response to Government's Growth* (Washington, DC: Brookings Institution, 1983).
6. The motive behind requirements for consumer representation in federal health planning programs starting with comprehensive health planning was to break the hold of providers on existing process. Theodore R. Marmor and James A. Morone, "Representing Consumer Interests: Imbalanced Markets, Health Planning, and the HSAs," *Milbank Memorial Fund Quarterly* 58 (1980): 125–65.
7. Marmor and Morone, "Representing Consumer Interests."
8. The classic statements of this point, in Aristotle's *Politics* and John Stuart Mill's *Considerations on Representative Government*, stress both goodness of policy and good educative effect on citizens. In our own time, conservatives (Michael Oakeshott, for example) and radical democrats (Michael Walzer, for example) share this outlook. For most of us, liberal individualism gets in the way of an appreciation of community.
9. Alexis de Tocqueville's 1835 account of the political advantages of the American states as administrative units is reconstructed in a provocative way by Martin Diamond in "Ethics and Politics: The American Way." In Robert H. Horwitz, ed., *The Moral Foundations of the American Republic* (Charlottesville, VA: University Press of Virginia, 1977), pp. 39–72. S.H. Beer takes a similar point of view in "A Political Scientist Looks at Fiscal Federalism." In Warren Oates, ed., *The Political Economy of Fiscal Federalism* (Lexington, MA: Lexington Books, 1977).
10. In addition, the federal government is arguably too large to undertake the planning that we advocate. Moreover, the states already have analogous programs, like CoN and tax-exempt bonding authority. The history of P.L. 93-641 has been one of the consolidation of power in state government at the expense of the HSAs.
11. Herbert Kaufman, "Emerging Conflicts in the Doctrines of Public Administration," *American Political Science Review* 50 (December 1956): 1057–73. See also Kaufman's "Reflections on Administrative Reorganization." In Joseph A. Pechman, ed., *Setting National Priorities: The 1978 Budget* (Washington, DC: Brookings Institution, 1977); and James G. March and Johan P. Olson, "What Administrative Reorganization Tells Us about Governing," *American Political Science Review* 77 (June 1983): 281–96.
12. This is the classic rationale for commissions at the federal level. Historically, the establishment of the independent regulatory commissions rested less on sound logic (that there were certain especially sensitive matters over which experts should be given leave to act autonomously from "politics") than on a decision favoring some actions and constituencies over others in this fashion.

From the beginning there have been cogent reasons for abolishing the independent commissions.

13. The results, in recent years, have been neglect of public works, artificially low water and sewer rates, and stalemate with federal regulators. Litigation has finally changed the situation, and the state legislature has now created a Water Resources Authority. The authority's staff recently drew sharp criticism for proposing a 75 percent increase in the combined water and sewer rates charged to the 60 member cities and towns. The steep rate hikes are said to be necessary to bring the system up to date and to meet pollution control standards. *Boston Globe* (March 19, 1986): 17.
14. For an early account of this organization, see Basil J.F. Mott, *Anatomy of a Coordinating Council* (Pittsburgh: University of Pittsburgh Press, 1968).
15. Michael Lipsky and Morris Lounds, "Citizen Participation and Health Care: Problems of Government Induced Participation," *Journal of Health Politics, Policy and Law* 1 (Spring 1976): 85–111; Barry Checkoway, ed., *Citizens and Health Care: Participation and Planning for Social Change* (New York: Pergamon Press, 1981).
16. Robert Caro, *The Power Broker: Robert Moses and the Fall of New York* (New York: Vintage Books, 1974), p. 16.
17. Ibid.
18. Martha Wagner Weinberg, *Managing the State* (Cambridge: MIT Press, 1977), p. 153.
19. Ibid., p. 152.
20. Ibid., p. 156f.
21. As we noted previously, the need to be responsive to private financial markets is part of the capital problem in health care.
22. Massachusetts has a Health and Educational Facilities Authority: "The Authority assists not-for-profit hospitals, health maintenance institutions, colleges, universities, other institutions of higher education, cultural institutions and schools for the handicapped in financing and refinancing capital projects and equipment purchases at the least possible cost." Tax-exempt bonding authority is the vehicle. Savings in costs of financing "can then be passed on in the form of reduced expenses for health care and lower tuition to students." Massachusetts Health and Educational Facilities Authority, *Annual Report*, 1986. This packaging of benefits would be hard to beat.
23. In Massachusetts, the Senate Committee on Ways and Means recently noted that many of the commonwealth's dozens of authorities issue tax-free municipal bonds with a revenue source pledged to their repayment. "While these debt instruments are not backed by the full faith and credit of the Commonwealth, the state is generally considered to be responsible for these obligations if the authorities cannot meet the repayment terms. In some cases, the state has made a 'contract' to repay the bonds. Sometimes, the state has a 'contingent' obligation by statute. However, even if there is no explicit state commitment to the authorities' bond holders, the need to protect the state's bond rating would probably force it to assist other entities in financial difficulties." Commonwealth of Massachusetts, Senate Committee on Ways and Means, "State Authorities: The Fourth Branch of Government" (xerographic copy, no. date).
24. Ibid.
25. Edward Banfield and James Q. Wilson, *City Politics* (Cambridge, MA: Harvard University Press and MIT Press, 1963), p. 84; also Andrew W. Nichols, "A

New Approach to Public Sector Involvement: The Health Service District," *Journal of Public Health Policy* (June 1980): 121–40.

26. "Good government," while sometimes more efficient than the older style, is often not very interesting to ordinary citizens. Civic loyalties provide weaker incentives, in ordinary circumstances at least, than do concentrated benefits and costs. For recent discussions of how policy making might profit from strengthened civic ties and local action, see Benjamin Barber, *Strong Democracy* (Berkeley and Los Angeles: University of California Press, 1984); and Robert Reich, "Public Administration and Public Deliberation: An Interpretative Essay," *Yale Law Journal* 94 (June 1985): 1617–41.
27. Edward Banfield, *Political Influence* (New York: Free Press of Glencoe, 1963); Caro, *The Power Broker.*
28. In the original statement of American pluralism (*The Federalist* #10) there is still this concern with deliberation about the "permanent interest" of the community. *The Federalist* assumes that the Senate will be the deliberative body. In our day, deliberation is more readily associated with the judicial process, or (like statesmanship) it is a ceremonial term reserved for democratic holy days.
29. It is more than that if the CHIB also controls some operating money, as part of a bad debt and free care program, for example.
30. There is a good counterargument, however. "Mirror representation" makes it harder to freeze out certain players altogether.

Peter Aranson & Peter Ordeshook, [illegible] The Health Service [illegible] Journal of [illegible] [illegible], 121-40.

26 "Good government" while sometimes more efficient than the alternative is often not very interesting to citizens, who typically have other private projects. [illegible] in ordinary circumstances at least, their more immediate concerns [illegible]

[illegible] and local action, see [illegible] (Berkeley and Los Angeles: University of California Press, [illegible]), and Robert Reich, "Public Administration and Public Deliberation: An Interpretive Essay," Yale Law Journal 94 (June 1985): [illegible]

27 Edward Banfield, Political Influence (New York: The Free Press of Glencoe, [illegible]).

Cato [illegible]

28 In the original statement of [illegible] argument [illegible] this concern with [illegible] about the common interest [illegible] The [illegible] assumption that the results will be the democratic body [illegible] ordinary deliberation [illegible] readily associated with the national process, [illegible] for democratic [illegible]

29 [illegible] is more than that [illegible] Hill [illegible]

[illegible]

30 There is a good [illegible] however, [illegible]

[illegible]

6.

The CHIB Proposal in Perspective

A RECAPITULATION

We began this book—as we began the research project that generated it—with the premise that capital funds and capital policy exert a far stronger long-run influence over health system development than most people, even most health capital specialists, recognize. Health institutions need capital to emerge and to survive. They adapt their behavior and, in many cases, even their values to please sources of capital. In so doing, they make key decisions about the availability, the technology, the affordability, and the productivity of health services. When, as in the United States in recent years, access to capital depends on the ability to sustain significant profits in a health financing environment that makes charity and community service unprofitable, the resulting incentives can be as regrettable as they are irresistible. Like the gravitational forces that at certain times of the year produce exceptionally low tides, the moon of capital access has lined up with the sun of day-to-day operational solvency to pull most organizations' attention down to the bottom line and away from compassion and service.[1]

This is the thought that began the book. We end the book rather differently, with a description of an institution that is concrete in its details and much broader than health capital in its potential scope of action. In principle, a CHIB could serve an entire "cooperative sector" and have capital projects as only one of many possible uses of its funds. Depending on the priorities of its creators, it could be used to do anything from purchasing special equipment for emergency medical services to managing a free-care reimbursement pool designed to increase access for the uninsured.

We moved from an initial appreciation of the importance of health capital to a design for an institutional complement to health care markets in general. Our definition of health capital widened to an encompassing notion of infrastructure that includes, in addition to buildings and equipment: institutions, programs, services, and—last but not least—the vital organizational and cultural capital that accumulates as communities make important strategic decisions democratically. We arrived at this broader conception by stages.

The history of policies affecting health capital presented in Chapters 1 and 3 showed that, although health capital policy, per se, is very important, it is the interaction between explicit health capital policy and the larger environment of health care financing, reimbursement, technology, and politics that creates the incentives that drive capital access and investment. Successful health capital policy therefore cannot be designed without considering this larger environment. In fact, if in the design of capital policy one pays attention to the final outcomes of health, equity, and efficiency, then it may be in its ability to ameliorate or provide a balance wheel to these environmental factors that health capital policy makes its greatest potential contribution. Yet, as Donald Cohodes persuasively reminds us, we cannot expect health capital policy alone to correct fundamental health system failures like the lack of access to care for the uninsured.[2] Even if modern hospitals and other health facilities were placed in every poor neighborhood and rural area, they could not be operated without labor, utilities, and supplies—inputs that can only be purchased with additional operating revenues. A broader policy and a more diverse distribution of resources are necessary to solve such problems.

To summarize, then, health capital policy has an important role to play, but to be fully effective this role must be coordinated and supplemented with other policies in a strategic fashion. What we lack at present, beyond the recognition that coordination is both missing and desirable, is an effective coordinating process. Such a process or mechanism need not take the form of an executive agency; it could be an economic market or a legislature or a referendum. The choice of mechanism depends on the nature of the larger environment. Because the dominant health system structure of the future seems likely to be market-driven, however, there is good reason to seek a nonmarket balance wheel.

We described in Chapter 2 how the health services environment seems to be evolving toward a much greater reliance on market mechanisms—toward a system of price and product competition among care management organizations and toward a more active involvement of business and labor in both purchasing and community planning.

Whether business and government will help structure emerging markets so that those markets can function fairly and effectively remains to be seen. As Alain Enthoven recently wrote, "A market made up of health care financing and delivery plans and individual consumers, without a carefully drawn set of rules to mitigate market failures, and without mediation by collective action on the demand side, cannot produce efficiency and equity."[3] Part of government's role (and the role of business and other community leaders) must be to write the rules and create the coalitions that can make markets effective. Another part of their job is to create alternative political mechanisms that can flexibly expand and contract their activities according to the extent to which markets fail to meet health needs and promote efficiency. No matter how carefully public and private leaders structure emerging markets, there will always be locations, populations, and services for which markets simply cannot do the job. What one learns by comparing political institutions to allocate health capital is that a mechanism capable of coping with market failure in health capital also establishes an excellent foundation from which to operate other market-compensating activities related to health.

Chapter 2 described three basic ways to meet the legitimate capital financing needs of health care delivery institutions: historical-cost reimbursement, market payment, and planned payment. Experiences recounted in Chapter 1 exposed the fatal flaws of cost-based capital reimbursement. Among other failings, cost-based reimbursement encourages waste and perpetuates the past at the expense of the future. Similarly, the Chapter 2 analysis of market payment's probable effects showed that market payment would be disastrous in the competitive environment of the future, at least for poor and rural communities, and for institutions with vital health and community service missions that the market cannot or will not support. These institutions and communities are left with planned payment as their only live option.

Is planned payment, the last remaining option, a viable one? Necessity may be the mother of invention, but not all inventions work. Can planned payment work? History describes a few brief successes: the early Hill-Burton program and voluntary health planning in a few cities. In addition, the city of Rochester's hospitals currently manage one kind of planned capital payment system, mentioned in Chapters 4 and 5 and described more fully in Appendix A. Appendix B describes a successful analogous institution from the realm of housing policy, the SHARP rental housing construction subsidy program in Massachusetts. There also have been failures. As a general rule, we have a far smaller body of proven theory to help design and predict the effects of political institu-

Exhibit 6-1
Future-Oriented Planned Payment Objectives

1. Maintain an efficient and accessible capital infrastructure and preserve society's investment in health capital.
2. Nurture and support essential services that existing markets cannot supply.
3. Identify and strengthen a cooperative sector within the health services industry.
4. Stimulate experimentation and innovation in the organization and delivery of services.
5. Strengthen and broaden community capacity to plan and act.
6. Preserve and promote competitive markets where they can be effective.

tions like planned payment than we have economic theory to tell us how markets will work. There are no guarantees.

Despite this uncertainty, we can expect the emerging market for managed care to support planned payment far more strongly than the old fee-for-service, historical-cost reimbursement environment did. The market itself will encourage operational efficiency, freeing capital policy from the task of curbing waste–a job it cannot accomplish–and creating the conditions of capital scarcity that give planned payment agencies leverage and popularity among their beneficiaries. In addition, we can through hindsight avoid the mistakes of past attempts. Experience suggests we should broaden the mission of a planned payment agency beyond an exclusive focus on health capital. It is this principle of institutional design that leads to the broader concept of a cooperative sector supported by a multipurpose subsidy allocation institution.

What other principles does history suggest? One principle is that better planned payment designs require realistic objectives that are appropriate to the environment in which they will function, in our case an emerging competitive world. We presented a list of future-oriented planned payment objectives in Chapter 2. We reiterate these objectives in Exhibit 6-1.

In Chapter 3, we also extracted a list of institutional design rules. Chapters 4 and 5 added to this list through the analysis of a variety of community health infrastructure bank design options. We summarize a selection of the more important design principles in Exhibit 6-2.

The importance of the guidelines presented in Exhibits 6-1 and 6-2 becomes apparent when one compares an institution built from them to a much differently organized–and, we would argue, largely ineffectual– program: certificate of need. A CHIB designed using these rules of thumb would not be just a CoN agency with more power and money. There is a world of difference between trying to regulate, with little real

Exhibit 6-2
Essential Principles of CHIB Design

1. Pool actual funds and give a single organization broad discretion, within a clear governing charter, to allocate them.
2. Charter the CHIB to fund several different classes of activity so as to create competing constituencies and stimulate vigorous, informed debate over community health investment strategies.
3. Provide operating subsidies and start-up assistance as well as capital support; recognize and require sweat equity where financial equity cannot be contributed; allocate funds by expected outcome rather than as insitutional or industry-specific entitlements.
4. Avoid formulas and encourage negotiation; dedicate subpools of funds to specific strategic purposes, and refuse to spend subpools until a group of excellent competing proposals are in hand.
5. Act as a facilitator, community organizer, and prudent buyer, not as a regulator.
6. Look to a tax on health delivery institution revenues, to appropriations from general revenues, or to a diversion of reimbursement payments as sources for major CHIB revenues; avoid attempts to leverage access to tax-exempt debt and similar soft-money techniques.
7. Stick to "hard" forms of resource distribution—grants, loans, and payments for services—and avoid the temptation to leverage current assets by pledging future revenues.
8. Organize the CHIB's top-down strategic planning process around the budgeting of outcome-oriented subpools of funds, and use requests for proposals to define desired programmatic outcomes; mandate ample opportunity for public participation in strategic planning.
9. Create a bottom-up process, separate from the strategic budgeting process, to award funds to applicants; make awards in infrequent batches rather than on a first-come, first-reviewed basis.
10. Design an organizational structure and create management systems that institutionalize a clear division between top-down strategic planning and bottom-up award decision making; create, in effect, two distinct suborganizations with different managers, different tasks, different processes, and different styles of discourse.
11. Make the CHIB a governmental entity ultimately accountable to an elected executive of general government, not to an assembly of special-interest representatives or a self-appointed community elite.
12. Unless compelling local circumstances dictate otherwise, make the CHIB a creature of state government accountable to the governor.
13. Although a governing commission or board seems desirable in order to secure attentive and well-informed governance and debate, resist the temptation to insulate this body completely from political influence and accountability.
14. Tailor each CHIB to local political institutions and culture; try to avoid imposing detailed structures or missions from Washington, D.C. or other distant states of mind.

authority or power, how independent institutions spend their own money, and managing a pool of funds on behalf of a state or a community. A CHIB differs still more from the National Health Planning and Resource Development Act's single-handed attempts to control cost inflation, democratize local health politics, and somehow rationalize an entire delivery system through regulation. The CHIB proposal's intention to allocate funds to projects and services that the market cannot provide is much more modest, far less intrusive, and significantly more likely to succeed if implemented.

PROSPECTS AND STRATEGIES FOR IMPLEMENTATION

This book's journey from a concern with health capital policy to a design for a community health infrastructure bank is a journey guided by the merits of the case. The CHIB is not an institution tailored from the outset primarily to please existing interests and political leaders. Similarly, we take stands on many details of institutional financing and design because these details are not merely technical; prior experience shows how crucial they can be to a CHIB's success. We hope a detailed proposal will provoke the debates that are necessary if viable CHIBs are to be developed. A vaguer presentation would offer broader banners under which to marshal political support, however.

Lasting institutions are rarely brought into the world by the wholesale adoption of detailed proposals. They emerge instead from negotiations among organized interests, negotiations that can succeed at those infrequent creative moments when the political and economic environment rewards collective action. At some of these moments, well-motivated and skillful negotiators with an appreciation of the merits and the details can turn probable failure into success. Our detailed proposal can help them. But any community's CHIB will be built from the ground up using elements to which organized interests can agree, not copied from this or any other book.

The question therefore arises of whether organized interests as we know them could ever give birth to a CHIB "in the wild." Can this book's vision, however sensible when captured on paper, be implemented? Can the idea take hold?

On the surface, the near-term chances for implementation might not seem great. Many leaders in the federal executive branch and in Congress, for example, advocate that the Medicare program use a system of flat-rate, market-style payment for capital. These advocates draw on philosophies and values that seem to reject—perhaps even to fear—

the processes of community planning and action that an effective CHIB would foster. Observers have been predicting for several years now that Congress will enact market payment. Can this bode well for CHIBs?

Actually, it can. As Chapter 4 mentions, market payment, by attempting to finance the capital needs of hospitals according to formulas that give each institution the same amount of money per equivalent case, breaks the traditional link between a hospital's "needs" and expenditures, on the one hand, and its capital payment, on the other. Aggregate capital-related payments to a state or an institution could be easily estimated under prospective payment—one merely needs to know aggregate hospital expenditures and apply whatever capital payment formula is in force. This makes it an easy technical problem to design a waiver application to divert a portion of the Medicare capital payment stream to finance a CHIB. It makes the political problem somewhat easier as well because no individual hospital will lose more revenues per case than any other, once prospective payment reaches equilibrium. And, because the bond between historical capital expenditures and capital payment will be broken, hospitals will be less inclined to regard capital payments as an individual institutional entitlement. They will be readier to see the merit in a capital allocation process managed by the community.

Predictions that Medicare will incorporate market payment may prove inaccurate. Although Congress approved the DRG payment system for Medicare operating costs in a matter of days, this very rapidity facilitated enactment. Capital payment reform proposals, by contrast, have been on the congressional agenda at least since 1983. Adversely affected regions and institutions have had ample time to identify themselves and to document and protest their losses. Proposals for market payment did not succeed in 1985, 1986, or 1987. Meanwhile, Congress found an easier way to meet its most pressing problem, the need to reduce the growth in Medicare expenditures and reduce the federal deficit: it simply legislates annual reductions in the percentage of historical capital costs that would be reimbursed. This solution, combining as it does the worst aspects of historical-cost reimbursement and market payment, cannot be applauded. But it does lead one to question whether the merits of a theoretically more proper structural reform will lead a large majority of market-minded congressmen to take the heat necessary to enact it, now that a less controversial way to reduce capital payments has been found.

In the longer run, however, the same result is likely whether Congress continues to impose reductions in historical-cost reimbursement or shifts to true prospective payment: there will be a call a few years hence for a new Hill-Burton program to address a newly discovered hospital obsolescence crisis. In the meantime, although failure to enact prospective payment for capital may erect slightly higher political hurdles for states that wish to experiment with CHIBs, experimentation will still be possible.

How possible depends to a significant extent on how vociferously wealthy hospitals and HMOs object to a diversion of a portion of their current capital payments to a CHIB, or to a tax on their revenues (paid ultimately by purchasers of health insurance). Implacable opposition is not a foregone conclusion. Hospitals in some areas of the United States were moving toward planned payment until they saw that Medicare and private insurance would allow them to act like independent businesses. The Rochester, New York hospitals practice planned payment now. Future economic realities may force hospitals in other cities and even HMOs to rethink their recent strategy of commercial individualism. Already, more and more hospitals are turning to philanthropy to support significant capital needs; wealthy hospitals may be a distinct minority in the near future. Moreover, in the final analysis, industry resistance hardly makes planned payment impossible. The decision to implement planned payment is a decision of the larger political community, of which providers of care constitute only one part. Florida, for example, enacted legislation that taxes hospital revenues to support free care, over the objection of many hospitals. Many well-off hospitals recognize the extent to which institutions serving poorer populations permit them to prosper. As the weaknesses in the emerging market system become clearer, and as political leadership changes, many states could find a CHIB attractive.

We have advanced the CHIB idea in the spirit of creative incrementalism, tailoring it to address the needs of, and to work well in, the likely market environments of the next few years. These markets may prove unpopular, though, and the nation may eventually find itself prepared to enact some sort of national health entitlement system that involves extensive public management and centralized capital budgeting. Many states are already debating programs that would fully entitle their residents to comprehensive access to health care services, using mechanisms such as bad debt and free care pools, expanded Medicaid programs, and voucher systems. Do CHIBs erect an impediment to such fundamental reforms, or can they facilitate them?

Legislatures might actually want to create CHIBs to manage some redistributional mechanisms. For example, CHIBs seem well-designed to manage the allocation of a free care and bad debt pool that evolves beyond a simple rule-driven transfer mechanism. Nevertheless, it is clear that comprehensive entitlement to health services would greatly reduce the downside risks associated with the reliance on markets to allocate health resources. A truly effective and equitable voucher system, for example, would place poor populations and their delivery institutions on a roughly equal footing with their counterparts in wealthier areas. The size of the cooperative sector could be dramatically reduced, although some need for nonmarket resource allocation of the kind CHIBs provide will always remain. CHIBs can be flexible in responding to future changes in health policy, however, including changes that *reduce* their scope of activity. Although the role for CHIBs might be less in some health policy futures, the creation of a CHIB now would not retard the achievement of these futures later.

A future health system that established universal entitlement through centralized budgeting also might reduce the CHIB's role as a plugger of underinvestment and underservice gaps. It would do so not by expanding the scope of the competitive sector but by reducing it and, conceivably, by making the competitive rather than the cooperative sector the secondary balance wheel. More even mixtures of markets and social management are also possible.[4] Any of these possibilities will require a well-developed political capacity for strategic resource allocation, a capacity that takes time to develop. CHIBs offer a vital testing ground and a possible institutional home for a variety of centralized management or contracting systems.

As can be said of the policy environments in which a CHIB might be asked to serve, the probability that CHIBs will disseminate widely depends in part on the evolution of basic national attitudes toward politics, markets, and other fundamental matters. After many decades of "dynamics without change"[5] in health care, ideology and economic relations are in flux. Attitudes are changing. We end the book with some reflections on these deeper questions.

POLITICS, MARKETS, AND THE PARALYSIS OF SKEPTICISM

At a fundamental level, this book is about the relative merits of political *versus* market mechanisms to distribute health resources. It is not an either-or choice, as we have stressed repeatedly—political structures are as essential to health resource allocation as market structures. But even people who accept the necessity of politics tend to minimize its role, thinking it a necessary evil rather than a positive good. For example, most advocates of population-based health services planning have tried over the years to substitute technical norms and the judgment of scientifically trained practitioners for democratic decision making. There is surprisingly intense distrust of democratic politics even among many individuals who simultaneously reject market allocation of health services.[6]

The avoidance of democratic politics leaves us with little experience in the creation of political institutions capable of allocating health resources. Similarly, we have little theory. Although academics pay enormous attention to the fine points of market structure and market failure, they have confirmed few rules to guide the design of institutions like community health planning organizations. This book offers guidelines, but the design of such institutions is a large task and the avoidance of politics tends to perpetuate itself in a perverse cycle: lack of experience and theory predisposes to failure, which justifies continued avoidance. The most common initial objection that managers of health delivery institutions raise to the CHIB proposal is that it would make the resource allocation process "too political," and the most common evidence they advance to prove this point is certificate of need, a political institution designed to fail. This is a Catch-22 situation not unlike the dilemma faced by the many countries governed by repressive military regimes – it is "too soon" for free elections and open political participation, but the national capacity for orderly democratic government atrophies with each passing day. To put the argument positively, democracy breeds democracy.

Apart from threats to existing interests and relationships, what may frighten persons of goodwill most about resource allocation by a CHIB or similar democratic mechanism is the lack of an external standard or *independent ground* by which its actions can be judged or regulated. Political decisions derive validity from the processes that create them, not from analysis or professional authority. (That they share this characteristic with markets, which also allocate according to process rather than science, seems not to allay our fear.) As Benjamin Barber says of democracy, of all the dilemmas facing it,

> that of uncertainty is the most poignant. Although politics is a realm of contestability and conflict where no independent ground can provide solutions, it is also a realm of inevitable decision and necessary action. The uncertainty that is part of the definition of politics vanishes the moment an action is taken. Yet measured against the uncertainty, the action must always appear somewhat fortuitous and contingent. . . . How can our human fate be the product of an experimental vision? How can individuals become committed to future lives that are no more than the inventions of a collective artifice? . . . How can we, once we choose a road to take, keep on the horizon of our common imagination all the roads not taken?[7]

Yet, as Barber also points out, "without decision and then action, the absence of an independent ground can only bring on the paralysis of skepticism."[8]

The solution to uncertainty can only be embodied in a flexible political institution capable of reflection and self-correction over time. Any such institution, including the CHIB we propose, must make its decisions visible and attract active community participation and debate. It can only do this if it makes decisions that are important and if it controls important resources. One cannot avoid the perils of politics by minimizing its range of action. As in baseball, one does not reach base in the major leagues by hoping for a walk, but by stepping up to the plate and swinging the bat.

A self-reflective and self-corrective CHIB must also remain accountable to the society it intends to serve. Accountability provides both the information for reflection and the prodding for correction. The reality of accountability, though, is more easily advocated than created. The reader is holding a symptom of the difficulty: throughout this book, we use the term *community* without providing a precise definition or a tested recipe. In New England, colonial town meetings succeeded so well at creating communities and serving them that they organized, fought, and institutionalized a revolution with remarkably little domestic social disruption given the pace of change. But direct democracy is hardly an option at the level of resource allocation we propose for the CHIB. Representative democracy limited to health (direct popular election of a CHIB board) also lacks promise, because members of the general public tend to lack both interest and expertise in health care delivery until disease incapacitates them for political participation. Similarly, we cannot reinstate the self-appointed coalitions of business and social elites who established planned payment during voluntary health planning's golden age. Most cities lack the cohesive economic structure and local ownership that allowed these groups to coalesce, and less populous areas lack the scale or the population density necessary to support many of the decisions that CHIBs ought to make. In any event, self-appointed elites are not sufficiently accountable to the whole community. Existing general government therefore offers the least troublesome base from which to define community. As Chapter 5 indicates, among the entities of general government that might define a CHIB's community, the best candidates are the states.

Are states communities? Not in the usual sense of the term—most of them are too large or too diverse. Still, as we point out in Chapter 5, states are the smallest unit of government that possesses established mechanisms for broad social choice and management. Are governors and state legislators accountable? Well, yes, via the peculiar institutions of campaign finance, party politics, legislative politics, and media-sensitive, low turn-out elections. There is much noise in the circuit of electoral accountability, however. Only a few of the community's loudest, simplest messages get through, and many of these reflect calculations of narrow advantage or thoughtless reaction rather than common interest and wisdom. It is because some of these loud and simple messages are among the more important ones, however—and because even these messages are likely to get lost in the noise of less democratic channels—that a CHIB must be accountable to elected political leaders.

Electoral accountability creates a background of simple but important messages against which a well-designed CHIB can tune in more subtle and complex signals. The CHIB we propose is also designed to tune out some insistent signals from the narrow interests that sometimes seem to dominate the deliberations of elected legislatures. In effect, the CHIB governing board constitutes a specialized legislature for health affairs, allocating resources with greater expertise, more information, more objectivity, and on a more responsive policy cycle than the general-purpose state legislature to which it ultimately is accountable. The CHIB can do this in part because, like the federal system created by the U.S. Constitution, it can balance off against each other the narrower forms of accountability and influence that would bias or capture its actions if its constituency were less diverse.

Eventually, just as decision and action drive away the paralysis of skepticism, we can expect CHIB activities to improve significantly the quality of communication from, and therefore of accountability to, the general public. As the current ascendency of "single-issue politics" shows, the electorate often sends its clearest messages in *reaction* to events and governmental action. The citizenry rarely takes the initiative to press for specific programs. When it does assert itself proactively its voice is organized by groups—often groups with something special to gain—and the subset of issues around which public opinion can be organized remains small in relation to the universe of issues citizens actually care about. We wait, for example, seemingly in vain for the public's overwhelming and long-standing support of health care entitlement to translate into a national health program. However, by allocating funds and making decisions that affect people's lives, CHIBs can establish a more active accountability by provoking reactive feedback.

Of course, reactive feedback can be as narrowly self-interested or as ignorant as legislative vote buying. But by framing decisions strategically, CHIBs can develop a more informed community, a community capable of resisting reactions that deserve only to be called reactionary. If, as we believe, CHIBs can be designed well enough to breed democracy, then society can build public management into health care with real enthusiasm and not solely because failed markets force it to do so. We can create institutions that, like the Constitution itself, will be defended for their integrity and their effectiveness even by individuals and groups who occasionally suffer as a result of their decisions.

NOTES

1. These tidal forces tug equally at not-for-profit, governmental, and investor-owned organizations. As the history of health capital policy presented in Chapter 1 makes clear, the fact that today's researchers have difficulty finding great differences in performance between proprietary and voluntary hospitals should not distract our attention from the real news, which is that for many years almost all hospitals have been very commercial enterprises.
2. Donald Cohodes, "Letter," *Health Affairs* (forthcoming).
3. Alain C. Enthoven, "Managed Competition in Health Care and the Unfinished Agenda," *Health Care Financing Review* (Annual Supplement, 1986): 105.
4. See, for instance, the recent proposal by Howard H. Hiatt in his *America's Health in the Balance: Choice or Change* (New York: Harper & Row, 1987).
5. The phrase is Robert Alford's, from his book *Health Care Politics: Ideologic and Interest Group Barriers to Reform* (Chicago: University of Chicago Press, 1975).
6. It is not a question of substituting some third alternative for both markets and politics, because there is no third alternative compatible with what might quaintly be called free government. The politics of expertise is still politics. There are no technical fixes for complex social decisions. Many persons and institutions do, however, share a stake in continuing to wink at the political and economic forces that underlie professional dominance. For physicians, this is true despite the emotional price they pay—and the scientific attack they must withstand—when they accept the roles of sole arbiter of medical reality and medicalizer of social problems that society currently lacks both the markets and the political institutions to resolve. Seen from this perspective, the distrust of democratic politics and of markets represents little more than a preference for current privileges bestowed and defended by a less than democratic form of politics.
7. Benjamin R. Barber, *Strong Democracy: Participatory Politics for a New Age* (Berkeley: University of California Press, 1984), pp. 258, 259.
8. Ibid., p. 258.

APPENDIX A.

The Rochester Area Hospitals' Corporation

Stephen R. Thomas

The Rochester Area Hospitals' Corporation (RAHC) is a nonprofit organization of nine hospitals, incorporated in July 1978. RAHC's Hospital Experimental Payment (HEP) program, begun in 1980 by contract with Rochester Blue Cross and government payers, was an unusual reimbursement mechanism, comparing favorably with other prospective payment systems intended to slow hospital cost inflation. But from the beginning RAHC aimed at more than cost containment. Other programs were developed. In 1985, with an extension of its contract with the principal payers, RAHC expanded the payment program (HEP-E) to provide a communitywide revenue cap on capital costs in addition to the earlier limit on revenues to cover operating expenses. At the same time, the hospitals agreed to the pooling of the differential costs associated with bad debts, charity service, medical education, and debt service. RAHC has task forces working on community health problems such as long-term care and mental health.

This appendix describes some of RAHC's experience in implementing these programs, placing the hospitals' efforts at cooperation in the context of health planning in Rochester and in the state of New York. The city and its industrial leadership are famous for voluntarism in

---

Information on the early implementation of HEP is, with some revisions, taken from "Note on the Hospital Experimental Payment Program of Rochester, New York," prepared originally by Catherine Lager under the supervision of Dr. Nancy M. Kane. That work was supported by a training grant from the Division of Associated Health Professions, grant number 5-DO4-AH01756, Harvard School of Public Health.

health planning. RAHC grew out of a rich tradition. So have Rochester Blue Cross/Blue Shield and the Finger Lakes Health Systems Agency. That tradition is not monolithic: conflicting appeals sometimes go out to the great examples from Rochester's past. Moreover, the financial, demographic, and regulatory environment in which RAHC's hospitals operate has been in continuous flux, and RAHC has had to adapt.

Within the Rochester community there are, not surprisingly, different viewpoints about what should be the future role and objectives of RAHC. These are differences about what the area's health and hospital care should be like in the future—about how existing plants should be used and about where new capital resources should be directed. Rochester is used to thinking of these as community issues. Even so, exactly how the community will decide is not yet settled. Government will have a role, but in Rochester—as elsewhere—public functions are performed by both governmental and nongovernmental entities, in an environment exhibiting both competition and cooperation, voluntary planning and regulation.

BACKGROUND: PLANNING IN ROCHESTER

Corporate interest in health care in Rochester has a long history. Several large companies locate their international headquarters in the city. Eastman Kodak is the largest employer, followed by Xerox, Bausch & Lomb, General Motors, and Rochester Products. Since Kodak and Xerox pay large portions of the health care costs in the area through employee benefits, both companies have in recent years strongly supported cost-containment efforts. Indeed, an informal group of civic-minded corporate officers who were also hospital board members helped form RAHC in the late 1970s. But health insurance in Rochester continued to exhibit corporate paternalism as well. At the insistence of board members from local businesses, Blue Cross of Rochester kept a community rating structure at a time when many plans were switching to more competitive pricing structures. Community rating means healthier groups of enrollees subsidize the premiums of the less healthy.[1]

But the tradition of corporate involvement in health care goes deeper than cost containment, and its original motives are hard to recognize in the current climate. In the 1930s, Kodak's management subscribed to a social outlook (traceable to the founder) that led them to focus on health care. Medical care might, with better organization, generate more spending and cease being an underfunded sector of the economy. As coordinators of services and managers of increased levels of funding, hospitals in particular could generate increased demand in the community and at the same time serve the needs of Kodak employees. Kodak was, moreover, in the forefront of the development of group medical practice and medical insurance.

After World War II, the Commonwealth Fund took a special interest in Rochester, finding there an opportunity to demonstrate the virtues of voluntary regionalization. Strong Memorial Hospital and the University of Rochester's medical school could be the center of gravity in a "natural hospital area." This was an altogether extragovernmental effort to show that medical care markets and medical technology had their own imperatives and could be properly organized with corporate and foundation leadership. In this way, the region could tap into a bigger pool of resources for the public good. The result was the Rochester Regional Hospital Council, a forerunner of the Rochester Area Hospitals' Corporation. As it turned out, the accomplishments of the regional council were more modest than originally intended, due largely to the availability of federal research and construction funds, which reduced the benefits of participation for local hospitals.

Marion Folsom was a primary force in developing early corporate involvement in Rochester health care. Folsom had attended the Harvard business school and settled in Rochester in the 1920s. As treasurer of Kodak, he was responsible for designing the company's first fringe benefit plan. With the coming of Blue Cross in the 1930s, Folsom enrolled Kodak employees. He was a member of the committee that developed the Social Security Act of 1935. Folsom served in the Eisenhower administration as secretary of the Department of Health, Education, and Welfare.

Returning to Rochester in 1960, Folsom was asked to chair a committee to raise money for new hospital construction. Folsom insisted that first a study be done to determine the region's bed need. This was a pioneering effort using community experts to assess the appropriateness of hospital resource use. The study concluded that Rochester's bed need was less than originally thought, and it marked another chapter in the history of corporation and community involvement in health planning. Rochester's historic, low bed-to-population ratio is credited largely to Folsom's efforts in this period.

THE FORMATION OF THE ROCHESTER AREA HOSPITALS' CORPORATION

As early as 1971 community leaders in Rochester considered the idea of global reimbursement, that is, paying for the health care of the entire community from a single limited pot. But it was not until the late

1970s that Rochester hospitals were ready to undertake a regional limit on spending. Perhaps because of prior planning and a much lower bed-to-population ratio than the rest of the state, Rochester hospitals were experiencing serious financial difficulties under the state of New York's reimbursement regulations. When, in 1977, a group of trustees consolidated the financial statements of all Rochester hospitals, they found that total operating deficits exceeded $6 million for that year.

Concurrently, in 1976, Blue Cross (with a grant from the Social Security Administration) undertook an ambitious project called MAXICAP to limit total spending for the nine-county Rochester/Finger Lakes region. The MAXICAP plan used the three subregions of the Finger Lakes Health Systems Agency, each of them called upon to develop a plan describing what the hospital system would look like in five years. Each hospital affected by the community plan was then supposed to create a hospital service plan delineating its long- and short-term goals for health care delivery. The two types of plan would be components of the overall health systems plan that the Finger Lakes HSA had to write in accordance with P.L. 93-641.

MAXICAP was never implemented. Several rural counties resisted the idea, and the Rochester hospitals were not enthusiastic about sharing control with dissimilar subregions, with the HSA, and with national Blue Cross. When the state Department of Health failed to approve MAXICAP, Rochester area hospitals supported instead the formation of a more locally controlled, experimental reimbursement system.

The Rochester Area Hospitals' Corporation had incorporated in July of 1978, and RAHC board members had participated in the discussions surrounding MAXICAP. In 1979, with the demise of the Blue Cross initiative, a new contract was developed among the Rochester hospitals, RAHC, and Rochester Blue Cross. In December 1979, the state of New York and the federal Health Care Financing Administration agreed to participate as payers, and the contract went into effect on January 1, 1980. (Exhibit A-1 describes the member hospitals.)

Rochester hospitals faced several incentives to join in the Hospital Experimental Payment program. Hospital boards and the business community were concerned about hospital financing, realizing that corporate and other private philanthropy would be hard-pressed to cover hospital operating deficits incurred under existing reimbursement. Rochester per diem hospital costs were relatively high due in part to a case mix of more seriously ill, shorter-stay patients than was the norm in the state. There was, moreover, little incentive to reduce costs below allowable rates because this would reduce succeeding years' revenues. Under HEP, in contrast, payers would reimburse a prospectively agreed-upon budget, trended forward each year for inflation; hospitals

Exhibit A-1
RAHC Member Hospitals, 1980

Strong Memorial—Operated by the University of Rochester as part of its Medical Center. 741 acute beds in 1980.

Rochester General—Teaching program affiliated with the University of Rochester; located in northern part of the city with 543 acute beds. Nonprofit hospital.

Genesee Hospital—University of Rochester teaching hospital near the downtown; 384 acute, 40 long-term care beds. Nonprofit.

St. Mary's Hospital—Part of the Daughters of Charity of St. Vincent de Paul. University of Rochester teaching hospital, located on west side; 298 acute beds. Extensive renovations.

Highland Hospital—Teaching affiliation with the University of Rochester; south side of Rochester, with 265 acute beds. Nonprofit.

Nicholas H. Noyes Memorial—Only hospital in Livingston County, serving a mostly rural area; nonprofit community hospital with 85 acute beds.

Monroe Community Hospital—Operated by Monroe County, with a teaching affiliation with the University of Rochester; 60 acute beds, 574 long-term care beds.

Park Ridge Hospital—Community hospital in suburban area of Monroe County; 194 beds, with emphasis on geriatric care.

Lakeside Memorial—Community hospital in Brockport, with 72 acute beds. Extensive renovations.

* *

University of Rochester—Like the other nine members of RAHC, the university has two seats on the board, including one filled by the dean of the medical school.

could retain any savings they achieved. In addition, the cost-based payers (Blue Cross, Medicare, Medicaid) agreed to reimburse for some costs not recognized under traditional reimbursement principles—such as working capital—and to provide a contingency fund.

Hospital board members took the initiative in forming RAHC. For them, the most pressing issue was the solvency of the hospital industry. But some influential observers in Rochester, particularly physicians, opposed the experimental payment plan, claiming that it was "part of a 'corporate conspiracy' designed to make profits for Kodak and Xerox." Industry representatives disagreed with this interpretation, pointing out that many Rochester companies strongly encouraged their employees to contribute time to community services in a variety of social organizations and that their primary concern was the financial viability and social responsiveness of those organizations. Savings in corporate health premiums were a continuing goal; the hospitals were expected to share with the payers the dollars remaining in the contingency fund at the end of the experiment.[2]

EARLY IMPLEMENTATION OF HEP

The new reimbursement program was in place on January 1, 1980, following a year of intensive negotiation and planning by RAHC staff and board members and the providers and payers. RAHC performed the monitoring, coordination, information systems development, and planning functions required by HEP.

HEP's cost principles and accounting methodology were quite similar to Medicare's. Thus hospital operating costs were reimbursed by cost-based third parties to the extent that their beneficiaries incurred the costs.

The HEP reimbursement methodology might be characterized as a "global budget"; that is, the total amount to be paid to participating hospitals was determined prospectively, by a trend (inflation) factor applied to a base year. The base year was 1978 for the 1980–84 fiscal years. Thus, a hospital received its historically based share of the prospective budget regardless of actual expenditures for a period of five years at least.

All of the cost-based payers (Medicare, Medicaid, and Blue Cross) participated in HEP. Charge payers (roughly 10 percent to 15 percent of total premiums) did not. If revenues from these charge payers caused a hospital to exceed its budgeted allowable revenues, then the hospital had to turn over the excess to RAHC's contingency fund. This fund, a departure from the usual Medicare principles, was funded by third-party payers in an amount equal to 2 percent of each hospital's final allowable cost each year. Contributions to the contingency fund amounted to around $8 million per year.

Reimbursement for volume increases, operating costs of CoN-approved capital projects, and other incremental expenses were limited to amounts available in the contingency fund.[3] Half the fund was available for volume and the incremental operating costs (excluding interest and depreciation) associated with capital projects. All expenditures from this fund required approval of the RAHC board. In the ensuing negotiations between RAHC and individual hospitals regarding use of the "community's" contingency fund, the capital-related operating expenses (depreciation and interest) were broken down into two categories. The first, covering building and fixed equipment depreciation expense, was adjusted for increases and reimbursed in full within the HEP formula. For replacement of major movable equipment, there was no adjustment beyond that permitted by the trend (inflation) factor applied to base-year, major movable depreciation expense. CoN-related incremental operating expenses were carefully reviewed on their merits and required board approval since they reduced the funds available to other member hospitals.

The contingency fund was also used to pay for the development of a data base combining all hospital inpatient medical records, billing, and cost information for communitywide planning. Certain relevant research projects undertaken by individual hospitals have also been supported. Eventually, incremental adjustments based on changes in case mix, medical practices, and new technology may be drawn from the contingency fund as well, subject to the 2 percent annual funding rate.

Control over the contingency fund provided RAHC with considerable influence over hospital volume and CoN-related spending. RAHC exerted this influence by means of negotiations with member hospitals, both before and after the submission of specific proposals. Since the RAHC board included trustees of all the member hospitals, the pressure to contain costs was exerted by peers, not by government or third parties directly. To be sure, local business interests were well positioned to represent their views on health care costs.

Structure and Functions

RAHC's board consisted of two trustees from each hospital and from the University of Rochester. Most work was done in committees reporting to the board. The committees often included people who were not on the board itself. The executive committee (board members only) was responsible for broad policy issues. The finance committee brought together the finance chairs from each of the hospital boards; they were usually also corporate financial officers. This committee reviewed all the hospitals' financial performance, interpreted financial policy, and examined the budgets of all hospitals, especially those of hospitals failing to live within HEP's "success measures." The medical advisory committee, including key physicians in the Rochester area, reviewed CoN applications and developed bed plans and other areawide planning projects. Additional committees formed around the hospitals' chief executive officers, chief financial officers, planning directors, nursing directors, and other managers. These committees promoted discussion of common problems and sought workable solutions.

RAHC coordinated hospital planning for the area, in part through review of CoN applications before they were sent on to the Finger Lakes HSA. The contingency fund, moreover, gave RAHC its own leverage over members' resource allocation decisions. According to one hospital participant, "RAHC can raise issues and get data that the HSA could not"—for example, the number of surgical procedures per capita by type of operation. Throughout RAHC's structure, at both the staff and the board level, there has been an emphasis on consensus building through prior consultation and negotiation. RAHC was an expression of the common interests of members of a confederation, all of whom recognized they were better off protecting a measure of local autonomy; hanging together was preferable to the alternative.

Planning issues with which RAHC has had to wrestle include formulating a service-by-service bed plan, developing general policy regarding new technology, and working toward resolving a cardiac surgery "crisis" and the "backup" problem associated with patients waiting for nursing home beds.

Besides these planning efforts and the distribution of the contingency fund, RAHC staff worked with member hospitals to develop a common "language"—a management information and reimbursement system expressed in terms that physicians, managers, trustees, and RAHC staff could all use. Costs would have to be a joint responsibility, and that would take common understanding. In due course, RAHC accumulated data on diagnosis-related group utilization and cost, by hospital.

The uniform financial reports generated by RAHC provided hospital managers with departmental cost comparisons (to other RAHC member hospitals and, at the outset of the experiment, to a set of Maryland hospitals) that were intended to help them pinpoint areas for potential cost savings. Much of the early cost cutting was done in overhead areas, though there were some efforts on the clinical side.

Here are two reactions, from an administrator and a physician, to the ensuing clinical reports.

> CEO: The clinical data reports are good for getting "the big picture" across to the Board; they facilitate Board and medical staff discussion. Since the data base is two years old, it doesn't generate an action plan. The data have helped to create an open environment and to contradict some myths. But the experiment's key achievement is the relationship that has been built up among the medical staff, the Board, and RAHC.

> MD: Rapid cost rises are in three major areas: lab, radiology, and pharmacy. We are getting each doctor to look at his own data and compare his DRG performance with other RAHC doctors, the nation, region, etc. It's an educational program. . . . We don't have standards of care yet so it is hard to interpret the meaningfulness of the data. Physician behavior hasn't been altered much yet on a daily basis.

A common fund of information promoted discussion and formed the basis of negotiations among professional staffs and member hospitals. As one trustee explained:

> It is hard to get away from tinges of parochialism, but the information and meetings help. Any individual hospital is treated as though it were one unit in a multi-unit company; it could be a plant in France under Kodak. RAHC tries to work with the unit in the same way that a corporate staff person would; that is, with the authority only to cajole and consult.

Chief financial officers and other administrators felt that HEP made their jobs easier. Payment predictability facilitated budgeting, reduced the guesswork traditionally associated with hospital management, and gave management leverage to resist spending.

While some physicians felt HEP imposed an "extra layer of bureaucracy on the hospital system," many others believed that the real achievement had been in getting trustees, managers, and doctors in the same room to discuss medical resource allocation.

Cost Savings: Examples

Administrative costs. One hospital achieved cost savings by carefully analyzing its administrative procedures and inviting employee suggestions. Some steps were as follows:

- Hiring freezes and intensive review of every position in the hospital
- Adjustment of salaries to communitywide norms for new positions
- Termination of "automatic" salary increases in favor of awarding merit increases at management discretion
- Creation of an internal audit process
- Increasing deductibles on malpractice insurance and self-funding the deductible, over time
- Elimination of extra supply costs in the housekeeping department by curtailing the use of disposables
- Introduction of a career ladder for nurses at one hospital and basing promotions on job performance and experience, not solely on educational background

Administrative change also appeared in clinical areas. Operating rooms were used more efficiently at one hospital after RAHC's analysis showed that operating room costs were out of line compared to other institutions. The vice president for nursing discovered that 42 percent of the hospital's operating room time was wasted because of a system of "block booking" for one surgical service. The hospital's board instructed nursing to "clean it up." Blocks of unused time were eliminated; rescheduling reduced overtime wages for support staff. Despite physician resistance and press controversy, the change stuck.

Rochester began to see new practices to deal with the "backup" of elderly patients, and the cost inefficiencies resulting from that backup. One such innovation is a "geriatric screening project" operating out of an emergency room. Many elderly persons were brought in by their exhausted families with minor problems, then "regressed" to a more dependent state so that they could not be discharged back home. The project identified families likely to exhibit "caregiver burnout." Clinical people sent visiting nurses to the homes to give the families support and to reduce the frequency of more costly hospital admissions.

Another RAHC-sponsored project was the geriatric inpatient demonstration unit. The 16-bed unit served acute episodes in chronically ill patients 70 years or older who otherwise would backup in the hospital. Unit staff concentrated on the social implications of chronic illness. Families had to agree to participate in eight hours of patient care per week. Length of stay in the unit could not exceed 45 days. Thereafter, the unit arranged for care at home.

Both projects were supported by the RAHC contingency fund.

Changes in physician medical practice. In the early years, according to one chief executive officer, HEP "only scratched the surface of the heart of the experiment–changing physician behavior [in regard to resource use]." Clinical chiefs and senior medical staff were aware of the experiment, but ordinary practitioners were not greatly affected.

Several participants expressed concern that even the five-year duration of the HEP experiment might not provide enough time to change practice patterns. The way to influence physicians, many felt, was to change the medical school curriculum. Others said that while there was "genuine curiosity" on the part of practicing physicians about appropriate modes of practice, no one has come up with the "right set of incentives" to get physicians to change their ways.

Despite the incentive created by HEP to reduce utilization of hospital services, physicians in teaching hospitals still faced a strong inducement to maintain or increase services that generated professional fees to support teaching and specialty consultant services. As other sources of funds for teaching and research diminish, especially support from the federal government, hospitals and their affiliated medical schools would have only patient revenues for salaries associated with teaching. If a drop in ancillary or other service usage resulted in a drop in hospital-based physician fees, this would mean a drop in the dean's discretionary fund that supported salaried physicians.

In the initial period of implementation, medical directors were uncertain just how to use DRG profiles to promote changes in practice patterns. The data might be presented to clinical chiefs who might then personally discuss clinical aberrations with specific physician outliers. One hospital used a diplomatic approach, presenting data at grand rounds on utilization and length of stay. Sometimes copies of patient bills were distributed. A second hospital formed an "MD task force" and directed it to "figure out how to change physician behavior." One chief financial officer approved a salary increase for a cardiologist, but made the increase contingent on the physician's writing a letter saying how he would go about limiting the use of electrocardiograms in the hospital.

Other Issues

Midway through the experiment, efforts were under way at RAHC to develop a DRG-based adjustment to incremental costs, so that changes in case mix could be accommodated. Meanwhile, chief financial officers and trustees were concerned about the rising costs of high technology and seriously ill patients.

A hospital board decided that one of its strongest specialty services had become so expensive due to technological changes that it capped the service's growth. New technology in cataract surgery, hyperalimentation, and cardiac pacemakers, for instance, increased supply costs faster than the trend factor allowed. Ambulatory surgery was performed for a greater proportion of the less complex cases, but the remaining inpatient surgery required more intensive resource use. As the base year receded in time, noticeable financial constraints could be expected.

Moreover, when 1978 was designated the base year, there were no adjustments (to reflect hospitals' relative efficiency or appropriateness of services) in that year's actual costs; accordingly, the HEP system gave an advantage to those institutions whose base year was fat relative to the base years of other RAHC members—or so some local hospital staff said. Some people wondered whether a fairer base year that disallowed or penalized inefficiencies would encourage better systemwide performance. Of course, this kind of argument could be interminable.

RAHC rested on the premise that strong corporate involvement and a businesslike approach to hospital management were good for Rochester. On the other hand, while RAHC was the envy of other areas of the country, the reduced involvement of the public by way of the HSA or the state was sometimes debated locally. RAHC staff sought informal ways to defuse this concern. Some corporate members and hospital managers thought everyone was better off with lessened public intervention. As one trustee put it, government implied "a benevolent dictatorship by uninvolved people."

Business coalitions in other parts of the country took an interest in the RAHC experiment. But as one seasoned hospital chief executive officer put it, "transportability [of HEP] depends on the nature of the business coalition. Many are formed just to wring their hands rather than try to work with the hospitals. The experiment is getting physicians, administrators, and trustees all in the same room, and making the issues understandable."

TRANSITION TO HEP-E

By the end of 1984, RAHC had achieved a great deal in meeting the objectives of the Hospital Experimental Payment program, which were to "control the rate of increase in hospital costs, improve the effectiveness of hospital services, and maintain or improve the solvency of productive hospitals." RAHC pointed with pride to the following specific accomplishments.

- From 1979 through 1983, the percentage increase in HEP hospitals' costs was 43.5 percent, compared to 47.2 percent in New York State and 76.3 percent for the United States as a whole.
- Per capita inpatient revenues for HEP hospitals in 1982 were $299, compared with $390 for New York State and $381 for the entire United States. The four-year (1978–82) percentage increase in this figure was 43 percent for HEP hospitals, 52 percent for New York State, and 72 percent for the United States.
- From 1979 through 1982 the Hospital Insurance Trust Fund costs per elder Medicare beneficiary in the Rochester Standard Metropolitan Statistical Area, when adjusted for variations in area wages and age and sex differences in the populations, declined from 89 percent to 71 percent of the United States average, making Rochester the lowest in the nation. Overall Medicare costs per Medicare elder during this period declined from 85 percent to 73 percent of the United States average.
- Hospital revenues (and RAHC received no grant funds from HCFA in connection with the demonstration program) have been devoted to a variety of research and development efforts sponsored by RAHC, including analyses of the correlation between nursing care costs and patient care requirements and patient classification systems such as DRGs, patterns of care of high cost

patients, organizational characteristics of hospitals under prospective payment, severity within DRGs, and patterns of care of particularly high-cost inpatient admissions.

– HEP was developed to improve a local hospital economy that had low historical rates of utilization, as shown by the following:

  – The number of beds, patient days, and discharges per 1,000 population in the two-county area (adjusted for patient migration) remained below regional, state, and national levels. The RAHC hospitals had 20.9 percent fewer beds per thousand than New York State and 24 percent fewer than the United States.

  – There were 25 percent fewer hospital days per thousand population in the RAHC area in 1982 than for New York State and 25 percent fewer than for the United States. HEP incentives resulted in a further 3 percent decrease in patient days per thousand from 1978 to 1983.

  – The discharge rate for the RAHC hospitals in 1982 was 25 percent lower than for New York State and 37 percent lower than the national rate.

In one key respect, the Hospital Experimental Payments program was limited – in RAHC's influence over the member hospitals' capital decisions. HEP had provided a communitywide revenue cap on operating expenses, but it did not originally cover capital costs as such. Early in the program, the RAHC staff had issued a set of criteria for hospitals to use in evaluating projects' merits under the capital approvals process. For all practical purposes, the criteria were ignored; the member hospitals continued to initiate full-scale requests.

Nevertheless, RAHC was not without influence over the determination-of-need process. CoN applications went before the RAHC board before going on to the Finger Lakes HSA. Although RAHC's imprimatur was not formally necessary, in fact no applications went forward without the RAHC board's approval. No hospital appealed to the state over the head, so to speak, of RAHC. Staff observed that projects were not actually turned down at the RAHC level; it just took time for behind-the-scenes negotiation, at the level of the hospital committees, to develop the desired consensus. The number and size of projects were typically scaled down in the early stages of the bargaining process. RAHC staff took responsibility for weeding out obvious nonstarters and trimming down and assigning priorities to the rest. One senior RAHC staff person observed that "the decision-making structure is such that 'informed choices' [were] made through the combined efforts of the RAHC staff, the CFOs, the CEO committee, a medical advisory committee, and the [RAHC] trustees." In this way, all the players learned how to schedule the community's calls on the limited resources available annually from the contingency fund.

Beginning in 1983, RAHC staff undertook discussions about extending HEP, with modifications, beyond its scheduled December 31, 1984 termination date.[4] RAHC proposed to extend HEP—the idea became known locally as HEP II or HEP-E—so as to provide for an annual capital authorization cap on increases in incremental capital and operating costs (including depreciation and interest) resulting from major certificate-of-need proposals. The HSA and RAHC would agree on an annual capital expenditures budget that would be used to judge the affordability of CoN proposals. In effect HEP's communitywide revenue cap on operating expenses would cover capital costs as well.

Another premise of the HEP extension was that the burden of responsibility for renovation costs, research and education, charity and bad debt, and the financial costs associated with CoN requests should be shared. Instead of building these costs directly into the hospitals' charge structure, RAHC proposed in effect a pool to spread risks and gain control over decisions affecting the community as a whole. RAHC staff could foresee the need to downsize hospitals to the tune of 20 percent to 25 percent of local bed capacity. In these circumstances, the Finger Lakes HSA agreed to the advantages of RAHC doing the internal "reconfiguring" of the Rochester hospital system. RAHC also expected member hospitals to experience changes in volume and case mix due to a sharp increase in HMO enrollment on the local scene.

These modifications in HEP required reworking the interface between RAHC and the Finger Lakes HSA, particularly with respect to the annual authorization cap and review of certificate-of-need proposals.

The parties involved agreed that there would be an annual limit—an authorization cap—on increases in capital and operating costs that would result from CoN proposals entailing more than $75,000 in annual incremental costs. Furthermore, by August 31, RAHC would develop and forward to the Finger Lakes HSA the proposed capital expenditures budgets for the coming two or more years. The HSA would review the budgets by November 30. Once approved, the annual budget would be one of the primary considerations on which RAHC would make its CoN recommendations to the Finger Lakes HSA, and on which the Finger Lakes HSA would make its recommendations to the state. Major CoN proposals to be funded within the annual capital limit would include those projects involving: significant expansion of existing services, addition of new services, major construction, major renovation, fixed equipment, or changes in licensed bed capacity.

Under the HEP extension, the capital authorization cap was a limit on the increases in costs of approved CoN projects. That limit was set at 1 percent of the hospitals' allowable cost base per year. That amounted to approximately $4 million per year or $12 million to $14 million over the three years of the new HEP contract. The capital cap applied to the entire three-year period, with some flexibility regarding the amount available in a given year: carry-forwards would be allowed.

In addition, hospitals, under the extension, would be reimbursed price-level depreciation for movable equipment rather than trended historical depreciation as before. RAHC and its member hospitals agreed that trended historical depreciation reimbursement did not reflect the current replacement costs of assets and resulted in a deterioration of the hospital's equity fund. The amount of price-level depreciation paid would be based on assets owned or leased as of the end of 1984. Hospitals would be reimbursed for the replacement costs of current equipment. Therefore, no additional funds for equipment replacement would ordinarily come out of the overall community capital authorization cap. Financial responsibility for certain categories of CoN projects would, moreover, be the hospitals' own, not the community's. For these "minor" projects, the hospitals would receive .5 percent of their allowable cost base.

HCFA approval of the HEP extension came in the last week of December 1984, just before the extended program was to go into effect. This delayed settlement of some of the operational details, and RAHC did not develop a capital expenditures budget for 1985. In its absence, RAHC and the Finger Lakes HSA agreed to this interim procedure:

1. A recommendation from RAHC would be necessary for the CoN process to go forward on major projects, those drawing on the capital authorization cap. The Finger Lakes HSA would continue to receive CoN submissions from RAHC hospitals for minor projects and would not require an accompanying RAHC recommendation for action.
2. Although relative need decisions with a capital cap limit would not be made during 1985, the Finger Lakes HSA would want to know, in connection with a particular application, all other CoN applications that would potentially draw down on the community capital authorization cap during 1985. The essence, after all, of an annual capital expenditures budget is that it is a mechanism for determining priorities among applications within an overall limit.

3. RAHC would provide a summary of the capital cost of all projects likely to be reviewed during 1985, 1986, and 1987. (A preliminary and informal estimate showed a total of $13.9 million over the three-year period.)

IMPLEMENTING THE CAP

Hospital X, one of RAHC's nine members, takes particular pride in its low-cost, financially strong position among Rochester's hospitals. It is one of only eight hospitals in the state showing regular operating surpluses since 1978. The hospital's chief executive officer believes that the Hospital Experimental Payment program worked because RAHC recognized it was "in the business of running hospitals":

> RAHC is the hospitals, not the business coalition, [but] I'm afraid it's breaking apart a bit. This town is getting more competitive. . . . There are people who say [the hospitals] don't have enough capital, therefore we need stronger, central local control. I don't agree. All the risk ought to stay with the hospitals. If they fail, market forces will control. . . . If I screw up, I have to pay the consequences.

As a primary and secondary care hospital, Hospital X does not compete with Strong or Rochester General in "high-tech" areas like organ transplants. Areas of exception, however, are radiation therapy and oncology, where Hospital X has historically been distinguished and has a strong national and even international referral base. With the completion of a big renovation project in 1977, the hospital still had support services that needed upgrading, radiology among them.[5]

In the spring of 1983, Hospital X submitted a $24 million certificate-of-need application. The application included three main components: radiology (new space and new services), new space and modernization of the main kitchen and cafeteria, and expansion of ambulatory surgery. In deciding to file the application, board members were concerned about the price tag, especially the level of proposed new construction. The application would be subject to later revision; in any event all CoN applications were in limbo until, at the end of the year, the state lifted the moratorium on new construction. Meanwhile, the board retained Chi Systems of Ann Arbor, a consulting firm, to evaluate alternatives. In December 1984, Hospital X submitted a revised application with a total capital cost of $15.26 million (plus $11.27 million for refinancing existing debt).

This project was important to the hospital, and hospital leaders pushed for quick consideration of the proposal in early 1985. Hospital X feared that its financial well-being would be hostage to the Rochester community's growing concern over excess capacity. The "extension" of RAHC's Hospital Experimental Payment program was bound to quicken the hospital's concern since its proposal would be an early test of the new system.

RAHC's attention focused primarily on the radiology component of the application. This was the hard part: here was where RAHC and Hospital X felt the pressure of direct physician interests. Kitchens and ambulatory care were parts of the hospital's future as a hospital. But determining the scope of radiology services was about the kind of inpatient care Hospital X would deliver.

The RAHC board authorized a task force to evaluate Hospital X's proposal. There were four principal issues: (1) the need for the new services, (2) how to apportion financial responsibility for the project's components, (3) the equity contribution to require from the hospital, and (4) physician access. The task force decided to hire an outside expert to evaluate the radiology proposal. Meanwhile other committees of the board considered aspects of the proposal falling in their areas of special concern.

Need for New Services

Hospital X wanted new radiological equipment and space for two new services, mammography and digital angiography. But was there community need for them? The task force's consultant, Peter Cockshott, professor of radiology at McMaster University, thought not.

In his January 1985 report, Cockshott noted that the hospital proposed excessive space demands as well as excess equipment capacity. From a systemwide perspective, the case for the new services was weak. Digital angiography was available at Strong Memorial, Rochester General, and St. Mary's. Current scheduling problems would work themselves out in time. As for mammography, it was available at 14 other sites, all of them able to handle additional outpatient referrals. So Cockshott recommended against mammography and against the digital angiography service, urged the elimination of the proposed tomography room, but supported conventional angiography. Hospital X's existing equipment was outdated and "an acute care hospital doing neurosurgery and vascular surgery does need conventional angiography."[6]

But Rochester radiologists, this hospital and elsewhere, persuaded Cockshott that in addition to community need there was institutional need to consider. After he had a chance to get Hospital X's reaction to his initial report, Cockshott wrote as follows to RAHC staff.

> Radiology should not be made the scapegoat for cost containment. Radiology services respond to institutional demands from the *clinical programs*

> *and it is these that need to be scrutinized.* If the Rochester community has excess specialized radiology capacity it is because the clinical specialty units are numerous and dispersed. This is no doubt due to historical evolution—whether the distribution/maldistribution is appropriate is for [RAHC] to decide. If you wish to make an impact on costs it is to the clinical programs you must look. . . . My report based on a partial data base may not be wasted if it can focus attention on overall clinical programs and their siting. Certainly the *institutional justifications* for Radiology at [Hospital X], despite special pleading, do alter my views of their equipment requests (but not of space).[7]

That the appropriateness of Hospital X's proposal could not be judged by a radiologist alone was a point that the staff could certainly appreciate. Still, clinical programs as such were not pending before RAHC. A few days after receiving the consultant's letter, the task force noted that it had "serious concern over adding new services which are already available and represent excess capacity in the community." At the same time, it was "sensitive to the hospital's argument for institutional need for the proposed services given the clinical services that are already in place at [Hospital X]."[8]

Financial Responsibility

Of course, it was one thing to claim an institutional need, another to argue that a hospital's new state-of-the-art technology should be a community financial responsibility—that is, should be supported by RAHC's pooled capital resources. RAHC was, however, part of a process that tried to merge the two questions. Once the task force found that its consultant could not stand by his original recommendation, it found itself face to face with the key question that the hospital's proposal raised under the new program: the need for "criteria regarding determinations of community responsibility."[9] In the absence of such criteria by which the proposal could be authoritatively evaluated, RAHC wound up reassuring itself that perhaps the new services were not so important after all:

> the incremental annual costs for depreciation and interest for the two services under question are well under $100,000 and therefore would not represent a problem in terms of community affordability nor place the hospital at a significant financial risk if they could not fully recover these costs in a competitive environment.[10]

Hospital X's proposal carried with it a conception of how to define capital expenditures from a communitywide perspective. Obviously, the hospital had an interest in being generous in its interpretation of the community's stake in, and responsibility for, the project. But the hospital also had an interest in packaging a series of small renovation projects in one CoN "in order to trigger the threshold for potential community consideration." Only projects larger than $75,000 qualified for community funding.[11]

RAHC's administrative committee took note of a second feature of the overall project approval process, one that likewise encouraged "packaging." Experience indicated that "small projects don't get quick state attention." This implied that a large and technically complex project like Hospital X's would get higher priority on the state docket. Thus the linkage between the local capital cap and the CoN process would push RAHC quite hard. RAHC would necessarily find it hard to mesh its local objectives with a *rolling* approvals process at the state level.[12] On the one hand, said the administrative committee, "there was a general reluctance to intervene in a hospital's right to work with the state in developing an acceptable CoN application." On the other hand, local review of the application required a decision about the apportionment of hospital versus community financial responsibility. In making such a decision, said the committee, "it would be helpful to understand *other* obligations against the cap *and* to establish criteria for spending against the cap before a final decision is made on the [Hospital X] application."[13]

RAHC was perfectly well aware of the forecasting work required to manage its payment program, and it had developed a sophisticated capacity to do that work. But in light of the pressure to get a RAHC board decision so that the state could review the CoN in April, RAHC decided to proceed in a provisional way. The Finger Lakes HSA would be supplied with a "not-to-exceed dollar figure for community responsibility." That way, its review could go forward in line with the state schedule. Meanwhile, community financial support of the project might wind up lower: RAHC staff expected completion of "negotiations regarding the final community authorization figure" by the end of March.

The task force wanted to find a basis for accepting certain components of Hospital X's plan as a community financial responsibility; the rest would be the hospital's own obligation. The whole project would, of course, still go through CoN. The task force began by distinguishing between replacement and new equipment. This put the proposal in the context of the mechanics of reimbursements. We can summarize this way:

Some equipment requests represented replacement which should be paid for through the price level depreciation provision of the new version of HEP. This provision, we recall, replaced trended historical depreciation. The underlying idea was that reimbursement based on the latter leads to deterioration of a hospital's equity fund, and community resources should be used to prevent this. But since replacement costs were reimbursed this way, no additional funds for equipment replacement should in ordinary circumstances come out of the overall community capital authorization cap.[14] Proposed new equipment, the task force said, would have to be "further identified by item as to cost, function, and reasonableness [criterion in the CoN process] in order [for RAHC] to determine that all such equipment properly relates to the community's financial responsibility under the approved CoN configuration."[14] The task force wanted to separate new construction and renovation dictated by the "major programmatic thrust" of the CoN from "renovation projects not directly related to [its] underlying purpose," feeling that the hospital should take fiscal responsibility for the latter.

Equity Contribution

Differentiating community and hospital responsibility was not an all-or-nothing proposition. Even RAHC-funded components of projects should, under HEP, get an equity contribution from applicant hospitals themselves. The state guideline was 10 percent, and that was the task force's recommendation. Some members of the task force apparently wanted to set a higher figure, arguing that a larger equity requirement would force Hospital X's board to reconsider the amount of debt it would incur with its project. In the end, the RAHC board approved the 10 percent equity contribution, along with the task force's stipulation that RAHC's finance committee should approve the hospital's financing options. Moreover, the RAHC board prohibited the hospital from undertaking a communitywide capital campaign. "Quiet approaches" to benefactors as part of "ongoing development efforts" were permissible, the board felt, but "consideration should be given to adding any funds raised in this manner to the 10% hospital contribution in order to reduce the borrowing, where *cost is the community's financial responsibility.*"[15]

Physician Access

Certificate-of-need programs assess the need for capital expenditures and therefore affect the access of physicians to capital equipment. Turning down this request for new radiological services risked, according to the task force's consultant, making radiology "the scapegoat for cost containment." Hospital X's physicians brought its institutional need for the services to the attention of the consultant and to RAHC staff.

If capital decisions are (in part) clinical service–driven, then pooling capital resources requires pooling service provision. To downsize in a mutually agreeable fashion (in that sense, an equitable fashion), Roch-

Exhibit A-2
Issues for Consideration Regarding
Physician Access to Services at Limited Sites

1. There should be no barriers to appropriate patient access to needed medical and hospital services in the community.
2. Duplication of specialized services should be avoided unless there is clinical and/or cost justification for providing the service at unlimited sites instead of providing access to physicians at limited sites.
3. Planning for high cost and/or specialized new technology enhancements should take into account physician access as decisions are made regarding location of equipment and use protocols.
4. Certificate of Need applications to establish specialized services where it is in the community's interest to limit the number of hospital sites should address the issue of providing appropriate access to physicians in the community, which will be considered as the application progresses through the RAHC Certificate of Need review process.
5. The hospitals' boards must continue to be responsible for the evaluation and credentialing of physicians who seek privileges to specialized services.
6. Physician access to already established services within an institution may be limited by a lack of hospital resources.
7. Newly implemented specialized services which require a period of time to develop staff or specialized activities should establish a time table for expanding physician access to the services if they do not initially make the service available to community physicians.

Source: RAHC staff, prepared for the RAHC board, November 9, 1984.

ester hospitals will have to find a way to link capital decisions with the expectations of the clinical providers who help determine the systemwide need for services. But this is difficult, and some say it is a problem that RAHC, with its hospital-based board, is not well equipped to solve.

RAHC worked for a year to produce a document called "Issues for Consideration Regarding Physician Access to Services at Limited Sites" (Exhibit A-2). It poses the systemic extremes nicely: "duplication of specialized services should be avoided unless there is clinical and/or cost justification for providing the service at unlimited sites instead of providing access to physicians at limited sites." Avoiding duplication, creating a community medical care system, required creating a community of clinicians. This in turn meant breaking down the existing pattern of physician-hospital attachments. The incompleteness of "access to physicians at limited sites" is the flip side of "duplication of specialized services."

The RAHC document on physician access reads like a treaty, with a lawyerly attention to language that is precise and high-mindedly vague,

Exhibit A-3
Hospital X: Summary of Financial Responsibility as Approved by the RAHC Board of Directors

	CONSTRUCTION AND ACQUISITION COSTS	ANNUAL EXPENSE
Community responsibility		
Construction, demolition, and renovation	$6,900,000	$371,000*
Equipment	710,000	85,000†
Salaries and benefits		(37,000)
Other operating expense		72,000
TOTAL community responsibility	7,610,000	491,000
Hospital responsibility		
Construction, demolition, and renovation	895,000	69,000
Equipment	2,720,000	323,000‡
TOTAL hospital responsibility	3,615,000	392,000
TOTAL	$11,225,000	$883,000

*Includes $109,000 for radiology.
†Includes $76,000 for radiology.
‡Includes $286,000 for radiology.

Source: Minutes of RAHC board February 28, 1985.

as needed. As a voluntary confederation of hospitals, RAHC depends on treaties. It is not a unified system of resource allocation. Its principal purpose is to protect its members from the most likely (worse) alternative.

The Hospital X proposal was approved by the RAHC board. (Exhibit A-3 gives a cost breakdown showing the contributions of the several components.) At the same time, RAHC staff insisted that the proposal was in some respects a special case and not a precedent for the future operations of the pooled capital payment system. With respect to physician access, the proposal had the important effect of focusing the board's attention. The board noted that "the current lack of definition of guidelines pertaining to project eligibility" under the cap made it impossible to refuse additional services. At the same time, the board was on the alert for the longer-run implications of creating additional capacity in its hospital system, in light of its own (negotiated) access policy. One board member noted that "both physician and patient access can be provided for elsewhere in the system." But in the short run, this was more an intention than an accomplishment.

The distinction between a hospital's plan and community need focused attention on a proposal's eligibility for community financial support and gave RAHC a low profile. RAHC would not interfere in attempts by the member hospitals to increase their market shares and would only decide whether a specific proposal was eligible for a contribution from the capital pool. Whether a project was, in another sense, a community need—worthy of a certificate of need—was for the health systems agency to decide. But, as Rochester Blue Cross was quick to point out, the HEP-E contract required more of RAHC. It required more because the Rochester community stood to lose from competition among the hospitals. Moreover, from a community point of view (as interpreted by Blue Cross), RAHC should take care to avoid becoming simply the hospitals' advocate. The contract in fact required, Blue Cross said and the Finger Lakes HSA agreed, that *any* incremental expenses associated with new or expanded services be included in (i.e., drawn from) the capital cap. As RAHC must have expected, the Blue Cross interpretation eventually prevailed: RAHC's capital budget (presented for the first time in the spring of 1986) would include only those projects that reflected community need, and only projects in the capital budget would be reviewed by Finger Lakes.[16]

A CAPITAL EXPENDITURES BUDGET

The Finger Lakes HSA had, as already noted, agreed to conduct 1985 CoN reviews without a budget in place (a budget was called for by the HEP-E contract)—"provided that RAHC review of an application was complete and identified the capital costs which had been approved for drawdown on the community capital authorization cap."[17] By early 1986 RAHC still had no formalized capital budget; the HSA had grown impatient, and its board was prepared to force the issue by suspending the CoN review process.

The fact that RAHC left community need decisions to the Finger Lakes HSA and exempted some capital expenditures from the cap contributed to the problem. Several proposals for expanded cardiac catheterization capacity now brought the matter to a head. More important, it appeared that by 1987 demands on the capital budget would probably exceed the total amount available. This was new. RAHC would have to worry not only about whether a project was eligible for community funding but also about whether the community could afford the project.

Cardiac Catheterization Laboratories

In October 1985, the Finger Lakes HSA board adopted a needs assessment for cardiac diagnostic services that concluded there was no community need for more cardiac catheterization laboratories. Three new laboratories had been proposed: one at Hospital X, one at St. Mary's, and a second laboratory at Rochester General. There are currently two laboratories at Strong Memorial (one scheduled for replacement) and one at Rochester General.

Nevertheless, three months later RAHC told the Finger Lakes HSA that it would wait for the HSA's decision on two laboratories: "HEP-E funding of St. Mary's Hospital's and [Hospital X's] C of N applications . . . is dependent upon the HSA's determination of need for such cardiac catheterization laboratories." This announcement prompted a notably blunt reply from the Finger Lakes HSA: ". . . frankly I find it difficult to understand precisely what we are being requested to do."

In due course, RAHC and Blue Cross settled their differences over the HEP-E contract to the satisfaction of the Finger Lakes HSA. The CoN applications for new cardiac catheterization laboratories were withdrawn, at least for 1986; there was every reason to believe they would be resubmitted as part of RAHC's 1987 budget. Everyone expects the controversy over additional catheterization capacity to be especially heated. Said the chief executive officer of one interested hospital, "There's never been a sound definition of community need. . . . I understand Finger Lakes' definition. I don't understand RAHC's definition." This same administrator pointed out that he had tried in vain for five years to get privileges at the catheterization laboratories at Strong Memorial, to the point where his own physicians were impatient with him.

The Capital Budget

The HSA's temporary suspension of its review of RAHC projects was meant in part to prompt RAHC to produce a capital budget. For the first time, the dollar value of future projects (their incremental costs) exceeded the amount of money available. In prior years RAHC had had a surplus. Now there were going to be more projects than the capital budget could afford.

The budget document for 1985–86 was in essence a summary of decisions that RAHC and the Finger Lakes HSA had already made, and it included information about items that had not been funded. The budget was a model for what now had to be done prospectively.

Far from showing a surplus, the 1987 budget—in preparation in the fall of 1986—will require criteria for assigning priorities to projects.

RAHC does not yet have such criteria, and it is clear that they will not come from the Finger Lakes HSA. RAHC staff asked each of the standing committees to propose criteria, but not much came of that. Currently, a set of criteria developed by RAHC staff has been forwarded to the several committees for their review.

EPILOGUE: 1987

A major reason for the relative success of the Rochester experiment lies in the fact that the structure of influence in the Rochester Area Hospitals' Corporation accords with the structure of economic influence in the city. "Hospital reimbursement schemes," notes an observer of payment reform elsewhere, "invariably are enacted and sustained by political coalitions that possess very mixed motives."[18] Rochester's "coalition" antedated the payment program and had a history of involvement in the community's health care. There is in Rochester a health care community capable of looking after its interests in the face of unfavorable external policy. At the same time, cost containment was not the only motive behind the creation of HEP. Unlike Medicare's prospective payment system, Rochester's HEP imposed a cap without the prospect of cost shifting by individual hospitals. Negotiation and the contingency fund made "community need" more than an exhortation, and behind community need lies a RAHC board whose members represent one conception of the community.[19]

But there are signs of increased uncertainty ahead. RAHC's contract with the payers expires at the end of 1987, and changes in the state's regulatory and reimbursement mechanisms are in the offing. Genesee and Noyes hospitals no longer participate actively in RAHC, though at the insistence of the state commissioner of public health they continue to meet their obligations under the RAHC contract. A proposal from RAHC to organize the nine member hospitals into three multihospital systems apparently was the immediate cause of the two hospitals' pulling back.

RAHC's planning process has always generated a wealth of sophisticated and reliable information, on which the community of hospitals has come to depend. Moreover, the several committees through which the system operates provide many opportunities for signaling and testing prior to final negotiations and a series of dress rehearsals before final decision making by the RAHC board. By the time debate reaches the RAHC board for a decision, the issues have been clarified and, if possible, the terms of accommodation have been worked out. When no accommodation seems possible or desirable, the board has preferred to postpone a ruling, perhaps indefinitely, rather than impose a solution.

Early experience under HEP-E tells us something about the relationship between RAHC and the Finger Lakes HSA. The present accommodation between the two organizations is about how to reconcile the classic, standard-based planning process with a community frame of reference, disciplined by an annual all-payer cap. But in the broader sense, RAHC and the Finger Lakes HSA are both instruments for community cooperation. Some local observers worry that RAHC may be too narrowly devoted to hospital interests. Tensions about community need express deeper tensions about who speaks for the community. For now, it seems plain that RAHC is useful not only to the member hospitals themselves but also to payers and planners.

Finally, a word more about the Hospital X proposal. The heart of the issue in this early case was what line of business this hospital would be in. In the short run, the influence of the clinical department and the competitive position of the hospital proved to be decisive. The test for RAHC is whether this continues to be the frame of reference—or whether not only hospitals but also patients and physicians come to be, as it were, community property.

By 1987, the paramount issue facing RAHC and its member hospitals had become excess capacity, a quite different situation than the members confronted in 1980. Even though Hospital X remains, in strictly financial terms, a healthy institution, its chief executive officer finds his hospital vulnerable. There are influential people in the community who think this hospital's closing would be the best solution to Rochester's overbedding, and each of the other hospitals has in its favor a more compelling argument for remaining open: geographical location; close ties to community ethnic or religious groups; or university affiliation. Hospital X, like the other hospitals in the Rochester area, operates in an environment arranged so as not to reward financial strength above all. There are deep matters of principle at stake in reconciling competition with community cooperation, especially as the hospital industry in Rochester is forced to shrink. RAHC was not designed to solve every problem, and it may not be well positioned to help much with this one. The community of hospitals does not, after all, speak for the community as such.

NOTES

1. In the early 1980s, Blue Cross dominated the private health insurance market in Rochester. Hospital revenue mix by payer was: commercial, 10 percent to 15 percent; Blue Cross, 40 percent to 45 percent; Medicaid, 10 percent to 15 percent; and Medicare, 30 percent to 40 percent.

For historical material on Rochester, which we have found especially helpful, see Dena S. Puskin, "The Birth of Regional Health Planning in the Rochester Region: 1960–1969," unpublished paper, November 1972; also Andrew A. Sorensen and Ernest W. Saward, "An Alternative Approach to Hospital Cost Control: The Rochester Project," *Public Health Reports* 93 (July-August 1978): 311–18.

2. In the first year of the experiment, Blue Cross premiums, having remained steady for a number of years, rose more than had been projected in order to cover the additional cost elements and the change in payment mechanisms. The slowed rate of cost increase under HEP for the following years contrasted with other Blue Cross plans.
3. Inpatient volume increases were measured only by increased admissions and were reimbursed at 40 percent of the average cost per admission. This variable cost was allowed only if admissions increased beyond a 2 percent "corridor" (i.e., a volume increase that arguably did not contribute to total revenues). Outpatient volume had no corridor, and the reimbursement was 60 percent of the per visit cost.

   For a general discussion of the details of early implementation, see James A. Block, Donna I. Regenstreif, and Leonard J. Shute, 'Experimental Payments Program: It's Working," *Hospital Financial Management* (September 1981): 10–20.
4. This account of the HEP extension is taken from a memorandum from Claire Lovinski, executive director of the Finger Lakes HSA, to her executive committee, February 7, 1985; interviews with RAHC staff have also been helpful.
5. Hospital X offers a full range of inpatient and outpatient services and is a major affiliate of the University of Rochester School of Medicine and Dentistry. The hospital has residencies in family medicine, general medicine, obstetrics/gynecology, and general surgery. The hospital's occupancy rate fell from 87.9 percent to 78.1 percent between 1980 and 1984, while its beds increased slightly from 265 to 274.
6. W. Peter Cockshott, "Consultant's Report. Certificate of Need: [Hospital X] Renovation Project," January 29, 1985, p. 6.
7. W. Peter Cockshott to Sara Hartman, February 18, 1985.
8. Minutes of RAHC task force, February 26, 1985.
9. Minutes of RAHC administrative committee, February 15, 1985.
10. Minutes of RAHC task force, February 26, 1985.
11. This feature of the emerging system was an outgrowth of the arrangement negotiated between RAHC and the Finger Lakes HSA. Hospitals were thereby encouraged to prefer aggregating projects to claim a community financial responsibility, rather than disaggregating to try to avoid CoN.
12. Unlike the state CoN process, the local cap makes only a finite amount of capital available for community funding.
13. Minutes of RAHC administrative committee, February 15, 1985. Emphasis added.
14. Claire Lovinski to the Finger Lakes HSA executive committee, February 7, 1985.
15. Minutes of RAHC task force, February 26, 1985. Emphasis added.
16. Technically speaking, a hospital can still appeal to the state, but this would be tantamount to secession from RAHC. The decision on Hospital X's radiological service was adjusted to reflect this view of the contract.

17. Claire Lovinski to the Finger Lakes HSA executive committee, February 20, 1986.
18. Harvey M. Sapolsky, Richard Greene, and Sanford L. Weiner, "DRGs in Theory and in Practice," *Business and Health* (June 1986): 43–46.
19. For a friendly review of RAHC's accomplishments and prospects, see James A. Block, Donna I. Regenstreif, and Paul F. Griner, "A Community Hospital Payment Experiment Outperforms National Experience," *Journal of the American Medical Association* 257 (January 9, 1987): 193–97.

APPENDIX B.

An Incentive Approach to the Development of Rental Housing: The SHARP Program in Massachusetts

David W. Young and *Lynn B. Jenkins*

In many states the supply of rental housing is a matter of great concern for elected officials. The dual forces of increasing demand for single-family units by upper- and upper-middle income families, and the inability of many low- and middle-income individuals to pay market rental rates, has led many developers away from multifamily rental units into single-family dwellings and other more lucrative ventures, such as condominiums. State policy makers thus find themselves facing a politically unpalatable scenario in which rental housing needs outstrip the available supply. Unable to harness private developer interests, they are increasingly turning to the public housing approach as an alternative solution. Yet, since public housing carries with it a variety of undesirable social consequences, the preferred social option is generally considered to be some form of mixed-income rental housing. However, this choice requires new thinking about how to encourage developers to produce such housing when the market provides few incentives. The State Housing Assistance for Rental Production (SHARP) program, one of several programs under the auspices of the Massachusetts Housing Finance Agency (MHFA), has been designed to overcome many of the obstacles to the development of affordable, quality rental housing.

Our analysis of SHARP uses an organizational theoretic approach that rests on the concept of "fit," an approach that can be traced as far back as 1938, to Chester Barnard's seminal *Functions of the Executive.*[1] More recently, Likert,[2] Lawrence and Lorsch,[3] Dalton,[4] and Young[5] have addressed the concept. According to this approach, the attainment of a high level of performance in a complex organization requires achieving complementarity among the entity's separate elements. More specifically, a fit must be sought, not only among the internal organizational, planning, and control functions, but between the entire organization and the environment in which it operates. To assess how SHARP has attained its internal and external fit, we examine its workings in some detail.

BACKGROUND

The MHFA was created by a legislative mandate in 1966 for the purpose of increasing and improving the supply of standard housing for Massachusetts residents. The agency operates a variety of programs for homeowners and tenants, including mortgage assistance, loan arrangements, and interest subsidy payments for single- and multifamily housing, most of which pay particular attention to the needs of low-income, elderly, and other disadvantaged sectors of the population.

Organizationally, the agency is a semiautonomous branch of the state's Executive Office for Communities and Development (EOCD). It is divided into two functional units—one for multifamily programs and one for single-family programs—each of which has an advisory committee that assists it in portfolio management, program development, housing cost analysis, and other operational matters. Each of the committees comprises 15 members, who are appointed by the governor and represent the fields of mortgage and municipal finance, law, housing development, construction and management, city planning, and social work.

The agency's general board of directors is composed of nine community, housing, and financial representatives selected by the governor, including two cabinet secretaries. The board sets overall policy and has veto power over virtually all agency activities and decisions.

The MHFA staff consists of approximately 200 people, whose diverse backgrounds include careers in banking, management, housing, architecture, and real estate appraisal. An emphasis is placed on recruiting people with "real-world experience" and technical expertise in the agency's line of business.

In effect, then, the MHFA is a semiautonomous organization that functions according to its own internal operating procedures within a set of state parameters. Generally, the state's role is limited to the involvement of its representatives on the board of directors, although on occasion, when MHFA decisions could have an adverse impact on the state's financial obligations, the state has exercised some discretionary authority over agency operations.

The MHFA traditionally served as a channel less for state funds than for federal subsidies, including both the "236/Rent Supplement" and "Section 8" programs.[6] These programs provided what have been termed "deep" or generous subsidies and existed in an environment where cost concerns did not significantly interfere with development goals.

As political and financial support for these programs waned in the early 1980s, in an era of increasing construction costs and shrinking federal involvement in state affairs, the agency's role shifted. The MHFA was forced not only to develop alternative financing arrangements and to assume responsibility for projects remaining in the Section 8 "pipeline," but also to cope with the overspending and other programmatic inefficiencies that had developed. The impetus for the SHARP program came from the realization that without federal (HUD) assistance, no new rental housing—either low-income or market-rate—was being produced in Massachusetts. Indeed, in 1983–84 alone, there was a projected shortage of some 200,000 rental units in the state.

As a result of these concerns, the MHFA recognized the need to design an efficient program that would provide good-quality, affordable housing to its target groups in the absence of federal support. SHARP was established to respond to that need.

THE SHARP DESIGN

Central to the thinking of SHARP's creators was the desire to dispel the MHFA's politicized reputation and to install a fair, consistent system of project appraisal. Historically, under the HUD 236 program, financing for projects was loosely arranged, and allocations were generally made on a first-come, first-served basis. There were few formal guidelines used to weigh the need for, or financial viability of, individual projects; rather, projects that appeared to be sound were usually financed.

Although the political atmosphere changed somewhat under Section 8, this program also had some arbitrary qualities. Under its provisions, the federal government gave generous lump sums of money to the MHFA, and HUD exerted significant controls over the way in which the funds were spent. Thus, while the shrinkage of Section 8 exacerbated the MHFA's financial constraints, it also decreased HUD input into the agency's decision making. Nevertheless, without Section 8, it was clear that whatever rental housing program emerged would be substantially more risky than its predecessors, since it would depend largely upon the internal strengths of chosen developers and their projects, rather than on large federal subsidies. Therefore, as underwriter, the MHFA needed to be concerned about the extent to which projects were economically successful, which depended in large part on their ability to meet the demands of the market.

In light of the above considerations, both the MHFA and the EOCD agreed that SHARP should meet some basic criteria. Specifically, it should: (1) operate on the basis of competitive funding rounds, (2) require developers to put up more cash and assume greater financial risk than had been required of them under HUD assistance programs, (3) reserve at least 25 percent of the units for low-income tenants, and (4) incorporate incentives to use the smallest necessary amount of SHARP funds. There was less agreement, however, on the priority that should be given to the financial viability of projects as opposed to their social benefits. When the final specifications for the SHARP program were written, the EOCD accepted the MHFA's position that a project should first be financially sound before consideration is given to its social impact.

The Section 8 program had asked such questions as "What kinds of projects?" and "For whom?" The MHFA now refined the questions, asking "How should projects be distributed, geographically and in kind?" and "How should funds be allocated?" SHARP was designed to provide essential support, in the most efficient way possible, for rental projects that encouraged a mixture of income and social characteristics in their tenant populations. Its creators wanted to make the selection process open and fair and to solicit the participation and support of all involved—developers, legislators, and communities.

THE ROLE OF SUBSIDIES

The SHARP program is designed as a shallow subsidy to developments that could not be financed by the private sector alone. Shallow subsidies contrast with the deeper subsidies available to low-income housing projects under the Section 8 program. For example, whereas the Section 8 subsidy for some developments approached $8,000 to $9,000 per unit per year, the SHARP subsidy may provide $2,000 to $2,200 per unit. Despite the comparatively small size of its subsidies, however, SHARP frequently can make the difference between the financial success or failure of a project.

To determine the maximum SHARP subsidy for a given year, the

MHFA begins with the estimated cost of producing a rental unit (for example, a two-bedroom unit). It then calculates the cost to the developer of financing construction at market interest rates, and recalculates the amount at a 5 percent interest rate. SHARP provides the difference between the two figures. Since construction costs do not vary significantly across the state, the MHFA feels it can set standard levels of subsidization without placing any particular area at a disadvantage.

By reducing a developer's interest rate for project financing, SHARP lowers the effective cost of the mortgage loan, and, in so doing, lowers the cost-based rent for all units to a level that is more likely to be affordable by local residents. Additional state subsidies can then further lower the rent for the low-income units that the MHFA requires its developers to set aside. So, for example, if the cost of producing a unit requires an $800-per-month rent to support it, but the local market will support only $600 per month, SHARP assistance can lower the rent for all residents to $600 per month. Additional subsidies can then yield further reductions (to, say, $450 per month) for low-income tenants. Since many low-income families cannot afford even that reduced amount, state and federal rental payment subsidies may fill in the remainder.

An important and unique feature of the SHARP program is that the subsidy remains constant irrespective of costs. In many similar programs, higher construction costs result in higher levels of subsidy for the developer, so that there are no built-in incentives for cost containment and efficiency. By contrast, SHARP offers major financial benefits to developers who keep their costs down.

To prevent a situation in which developers cut corners excessively to keep their costs low, and then pocket the savings, the MHFA developed an extensive monitoring process to ensure that quality criteria are being met. Additionally, of course, developers are monitored by their market environments; if they attempt to cut costs too extensively, it is quite likely that they will find it difficult to rent their units. As a result, developers must be aware of what the local market will bear, and make certain that their projects are compatible with both the needs and financial circumstances of potential tenants.

It is important to note the sources of demand for rental housing in this context. Specifically, the need for rental housing subsidies exists independent of the 25 percent low-income component that SHARP includes in its criteria. That is, because of a mismatch between construction costs, financing costs, and market rental rates, even if developers provide only market-rate units—and no low-income units—they still are unable to build "affordable" rental housing. Thus, the SHARP subsidy encourages the development not only of low-income units but of rental units in general. As a result, since federal and state assistance programs guarantee rent for low-income tenants, a developer's concern lies primarily with marketing the remaining 75 percent of the units. Effectively, then, SHARP fills the gap between cost-based rent and attainable rent in a given market area.[7]

THE FINANCING PROCESS

In 1984, its first year of operation, SHARP received a $5 million appropriation from the state. This amount was increased to $13 million in 1985. In both years, the program supplemented its appropriation by raising funds through the sale of tax-exempt bonds to private investors. The agency then translates the low interest rates it *pays* to its investors into below-market interest rates it *charges* to developers.

Projects selected for financing are awarded interest-reduction subsidies for a maximum 15-year period, over which the subsidy is gradually diminished. Specific terms of both assistance and repayment are negotiated individually between the MHFA and the developer in accordance with the developer's projected cash flows. The subsidy is not a grant; it is a loan that must be repaid by the time that the project has been in operation for the 15 years.

While the MHFA can exert minimal pressure on a project once the loan has expired, developers are required, as part of the application process, to explain how the interests of low-income residents will be protected after the SHARP subsidy ends. For example, if a project is to be converted to condominiums, developers might arrange to help low-income tenants purchase their units, or retain them as reasonably priced rental units. Or the developer might transfer the units to the local housing authority at sale or refinancing. To the extent that it can do so, the MHFA encourages developers to incorporate such provisions into their initial financing agenda.

PROJECT SELECTION

SHARP selects projects according to a set of firmly established guidelines. Once each year there is a "competition" in which developers submit projects, vying with one another for SHARP assistance. Out of approximately 60 entries in the first competition, 23 developments were chosen; of 40 entries in the second competition, 13 were chosen.

Projects submitted to the competition are scored and ranked according to a complex set of criteria, shown in Exhibit B-1. In designing these criteria, the EOCD and the MHFA asked, "What are the critical elements

Exhibit B-1

SHARP Project Selection Criteria

After projects passed the set of initial threshold guidelines, they were competitively scored to determine how well they met certain policy objectives of the SHARP program. This review covered the following objectives:

A. Development Quality Goals: 10 points each, maximum of 50 points. Projects must score a minimum of 30 points and have an acceptable design score to remain in the competition.

1. Design—the quality of the proposed design, including life-cycle costs and the treatment of special environmental conditions.
2. Development Team—the record and capacity of the development team.
3. Site—the suitability of the proposed site for housing. The presence of or plans for necessary utilities and amenities. Zoning and site control.
4. Management—the prospective manageability of the development, the quality of the management plan, and the experience and capacity of the management agent.
5. Marketability—the likely ability of the units to be marketed at the proposed rents.

B. Overall Impact Goals: 10 points each, maximum of 40 points.

1. Community Impacts—projects with demonstrable impacts upon the community, in support of local policies. Such projects include those which would rehabilitate a critical building in a business district, encourage additional nearby development, or promote investment in a locally targeted revitalization district. Evidence of local support would include contributions to the project from the community. Projects should not encourage displacement. Projects would ideally increase the supply of affordable housing in areas suffering displacement.
2. Meet Housing Needs—projects which best meet the overall housing needs of communities in which they will be located (i.e., units of a certain size).
3. Affirmative Action—SHARP encourages developers to provide housing and job opportunities to minorities. Applications which provide vigorous affirmative action efforts, beyond the minimum requirements considered during the threshold review, will be given special preference.
4. Readiness to Move to Construction—the readiness of proposals to move quickly to construction. Evidence of readiness would include proper zoning for the proposal, advanced design documents, building permits.

C. Minimal SHARP Subsidy Goal: 10 points. Projects that require less than the maximum permitted amount of SHARP subsidy may earn up to 10 additional points. This criterion is consistent with a desire to generate the greatest level of housing production for the amount of SHARP funds authorized by the legislature.

Maximum Total Points = 100

After the projects are scored and ranked, the MHFA selects the highest-ranked projects to receive subsidy awards, subject to consideration of two additional program objectives. Some of the selected projects should complement efforts to revitalize specific urban neighborhoods, and there should be a reasonable distribution of selected projects throughout the state.

Following selection of a proposal for SHARP funding, its developer is invited to submit a full mortgage application for MHFA review. At this level of review, the technical acceptability of the project, the financial feasibility of the accepted loan, and the value and marketability of the completed housing are evaluated.

that make a project viable?" The resulting threshold requirements establish the minimum viability of the project, and a set of secondary criteria incorporate social and financial concerns. Gates and cross-checks have been established to assure that high-priority conditions are adequately met.

In the threshold evaluation, projects are assessed in terms of their acceptability as credit risks and real estate transactions. The threshold criteria include measures of (1) the quality of the project design, (2) the suitability of the site, (3) the experience record of the development team, (4) the qualifications of the management company, and (5) the marketability of the project.

Applications that pass the threshold review are distributed within the MHFA for more intensive evaluations in each of the agency's functional subdivisions. At this level of review, questions relate to community impact, ability to meet housing needs, affirmative action, and readiness to move to construction.

After the second level of review is complete, projects are ranked and their scores compared. Discrepancies among scores are assessed to ensure interrater reliability. For example, if a particular developer submitted four projects and received four different scores for the experience rating, either the scores are equalized or the reasons underlying the differences are documented. The developer may have proposed four different types of construction which require very different levels of experience. In addition to the departmental scoring, some of the MHFA senior management and selected board members visit all proposed sites to assess their apparent strengths and weaknesses.

Generally, senior management, board members, and the MHFA staff reach consensus with a good deal of negotiation, persuasion, and discussion. In disputed decisions, senior management can overrule the staff, and the board, in turn, can overrule senior management.

Developers are also permitted to challenge the scores they receive. As of the end of 1985, however, no developer had failed to agree with the agency's score after all appeals had been made. Agency executives attribute this success to the precision of the selection criteria, the quality of the staff, and the system's emphasis on fairness.

STRATEGY

SHARP came into existence because the commonwealth of Massachusetts believed that the free market for housing was not working adequately. Because the cost of construction had outdistanced market rental rates, no new rental housing was being built. One could argue that the free market simply had not had time to adjust to new cost pressures and that, given sufficient time, consumers would be willing to pay a higher portion of their incomes for housing. Developers would then have found it profitable, without assistance from the state, to build rental housing. The argument for SHARP's existence thus becomes more a social than an economic one. Specifically, the state intervened in the free market because it considered it important to provide citizens access to adequate housing at rental rates that did not exceed some "socially appropriate" percentage of their incomes.

Once the case for intervention had been made, however, SHARP still faced the difficult task of determining where and how to spend the scarce capital resources available. Here, the essential tasks became those of establishing a strategic orientation—a set of priorities—and selecting projects in accordance with that orientation. In SHARP's case the expressed goal is to achieve a distribution of "affordable" rental housing throughout the state that keeps pace with the population's needs.

Kenneth Andrews defined "strategy" in a business context as a company's "pattern of major objectives, purposes, or goals and essential policies and plans for achieving those goals, stated in such a way as to define what business the company is in or is to be in and the kind of company it is to be."[8]

SHARP's overall objective is quite basic: to increase the supply of all rental housing in the state, giving special consideration to the needs of low-income individuals. SHARP's policy for achieving this objective is to provide financial incentives for housing construction. By borrowing funds in the tax-exempt bond market to supplement its state budget allocation, SHARP can offer shallow subsidies to developers in the form of long-term (15-year), low-interest-rate loans.

SHARP's intervention in the housing market is thus relatively limited but extremely powerful. Since its financial incentives to developers have resulted in a relatively large number of proposals being submitted for each competition, SHARP's key task becomes that of selecting projects that are, first, financially viable and, second, socially beneficial.

Financial viability is sought via an interlocking network of incentives to developers. Because the SHARP subsidy is pegged to a per-unit cost and is fixed regardless of the *actual* cost of construction, developers have an incentive to build their projects at or below budget. Moreover, SHARP holds developers responsible for the overall financial success of their projects, including taking the risk for unoccupied units. Further, SHARP attempts to assure itself of the financial viability of a project at the time the project is considered for financing. It accomplishes this by means of its development quality goals (see Exhibit B-1), all of which are related to the question of financial viability. Finally, although most of its effort is directed toward the "front end," i.e., protecting itself from financial insecurity, SHARP nevertheless continues to monitor its projects once they are selected to be certain that they are meeting their proposed budgets and other criteria.

In short, SHARP is able to use some relatively minor financial investments in its projects as leverage to promote the production of housing that is affordable, produces an acceptable return for developers, and includes units for low-income renters. It appears as though all players win.

Clearly, any process that attempts to define a set of social priorities and superimpose them on a market driven by economic realities will encounter political influences. That SHARP appears to have mitigated, if not almost entirely avoided, these pressures certainly does not negate their existence. Indeed, it would appear that political influences have been muted in large part—and the organization's strategy reinforced—by the way in which SHARP was created. Specifically, the participation of key political actors in the early stages of program design encouraged their subsequent support for SHARP's organizational structure and management control system.

ORGANIZATIONAL STRUCTURE

The structure of the SHARP program includes a number of elements that seem to enhance its ability to perform in the desired way and to avoid undue political influence. In particular, the following organizational features appear to be important:

- The agency is a semiautonomous branch of the state government. This allows it to function without the same level of political pressure that could be applied to a state agency, while still retaining its accountability for decisions that affect the public.
- The MHFA operates under the aegis of a state agency—the Executive Office for Communities and Development—which creates a certain amount of healthy tension. This tension appeared most strikingly in the process for determining project selection criteria, where the EOCD's social goals were balanced against the MHFA's development quality (i.e., financial viability) goals.
- The MHFA board of directors is appointed by the governor and includes the appropriate cabinet-level secretaries, thereby assuring the governor of significant ongoing control over agency policy at the highest level.
- SHARP is part of one of two "functional units" of the MHFA—

multifamily housing and single-family housing–each of which is problem-oriented and each of which has its own advisory committee appointed by the governor. This structure allows the governor to retain a fair amount of control over agency policy and also to see to it that the policy is based on expert opinion in each functional area.

–Within each functional unit, SHARP has organized its staff into further functional divisions: design, mortgage, site, management. In each of these subdivision, SHARP's staff members are experts in the matters under their jurisdiction. Thus, it is difficult to question the agency's professional qualifications.

MANAGEMENT CONTROL SYSTEM

SHARP's management control system consists of essentially two elements or subsystems: the project-selection system and the project-implementation system. As Exhibit B-1 indicates, SHARP's project-selection system provides a direct link to the organization's strategy. This linkage, or fit, between the management control system and institutional strategy is an essential ingredient in the design of any organization.[9]

Three elements stand out in particular as reinforcements of the relationships between institutional strategy and the management control system, and among institutional strategy, the management control system, and the organizational structure. The first is the emphasis on financial viability. Despite the importance of being assured that the projects SHARP subsidizes are financially sound, not all participants in the design process agreed initially that financial criteria should be paramount in the project-selection system. Yet SHARP's strategy of limited subsidization is predicated on its borrowing in the tax-free bond market; its rate is highly dependent on its bond rating, and the bond rating in turn is directly linked to the financial success of its projects. To have a threshold review that placed only minimal emphasis on financial criteria would either result in consumption of extra resources in the review process (i.e., for those projects that are not financially viable) or would open the possibility of providing funding for financially unsound projects. Either outcome would work to SHARP's detriment.

The second element that reinforces the fit among strategy, structure, and the management control system is the involvement of senior management in two critical aspects of the project-selection system. First, since SHARP can expect that there will be political pressure to accept at least some unworkable projects, senior management, by gaining early knowledge of problem projects (i.e., projects that are financially unsound but have a high political investment), can preempt much of the pressure; this happened in at least one instance during the past two years. Second, by actually visiting all sites and personally assessing their quality, senior management is able to gain independent knowledge of this key element in the project-selection criteria; consequently, it maintains a degree of control over the staff's assessment that it otherwise would not have.

The third reinforcing feature is the absence of a "zero-sum game" among developers. Specifically, since SHARP depends on successful projects, it must assure itself that developers are not discouraged from entering the competition. By allowing developers to reapply if their proposed projects are not accepted, and by working with them to improve the quality of their projects, SHARP is able both to diffuse much of the political pressure that otherwise would accumulate and to improve the quality of its projects overall.

The link between the project *implementation* system and SHARP's strategy is principally illustrated in terms of SHARP's fixed subsidy and its ongoing monitoring of projects. Here again, the organization's limited financial resources—the fact that it is a shallow-subsidy program attempting to generate as many housing units as it can with a relatively small amount of funds—appears to have driven the design of the management control system. SHARP must be certain that its funds are used as efficiently as possible; the fixed subsidy is a key element in obtaining that assurance. Ongoing monitoring of projects reinforces this element by allowing SHARP to flag projects that are in trouble so that it can intervene when necessary. This activity, in turn, is reinforced by a hiring policy that assures the agency that its interventions will be made by individuals with respect in the housing community.

SUMMARY

With the great reduction in federal resources available for improving housing, many states and municipalities are attempting to fill the void. Most must develop programs involving shallow subsidies since available resources are limited. The two key determinants of success become the attraction of developers and the assurance that the developers are both effective and efficient in constructing housing units. The need to provide housing for lower-income families complicates this scenario.

In this regard, the SHARP program not only is a useful prototype because of its multifaceted strategy, but is a valuable example of the importance of relating strategy and organizational design. Indeed, if housing agencies are to be successful in redirecting limited financial resources and meeting the increasing demand for rental units, they must assure themselves that their various organizational elements—strategy, structure, and management control system—work in concert.

NOTES

1. Chester Barnard. *The Functions of the Executive* (Cambridge, MA: Harvard University Press, 1938).
2. Rensis Likert. *The Human Organization* (New York: McGraw-Hill, 1967).
3. Paul Lawrence and J.W. Lorsch. *Organization and Environment* (Homewood, IL: Richard D. Irwin, Inc., 1969).
4. Gene W. Dalton. "Motivation and Control in Organizations." In Gene W. Dalton and P. R. Lawrence, *Motivation and Control in Organizations* (Homewood, IL: Richard D. Irwin, Inc. and Dorsey Press, 1971).
5. David W. Young. "Administrative Theory and Administrative Systems: A Synthesis among Diverging Fields of Inquiry," *Accounting, Organizations and Society* 4, 3 (1979): 235–44.
6. Both "236" and "Section 8" were subsidy programs administered by the U.S. Department of Housing and Urban Development. They provided assistance to developers of rental housing particularly for low-income and elderly residents.
7. Cost-based rent is defined as the rent needed to support the mortgage loan and the operating costs of a project (administration and management, routine and preventive maintenance, utilities, insurance, security and real estate taxes). Attainable rent is defined as the maximum rate at which units can be rented in a given area.
8. Kenneth Andrews. *The Concept of Corporate Strategy* (Homewood, IL: Dow Jones-Irwin, Inc., 1971).
9. For additional details on this argument see Young, "Administrative Theory and Administrative Systems," pp. 235–44.

INDEX

T

U

V

W–Y

About the Authors

During the writing of this book, JONATHAN BETZ BROWN was Assistant Professor of Public Policy and Health Planning in the Department of Health Policy and Management at the Harvard University School of Public Health, and principal investigator of the Health Capital Project from which the book emerged. In addition to the Health Capital Project, Dr. Brown worked with the Harvard Community Health Plan and Harvard's Institute for Health Research on the development of performance measures for managed care systems, and with a variety of governmental and public organizations on policy and management topics. Dr. Brown, a native of Portland, Oregon, graduated from the Public Policy Program, a professional master's degree program of Harvard's John F. Kennedy School of Government, in 1976. In 1981, he received a Ph.D. in public policy through the Committee on Higher Degrees in Public Policy of the Harvard Graduate School of Arts and Sciences. In 1987, Dr. Brown returned to Portland to join the Kaiser-Permanente Center for Health Research, where he continues his research in performance measurement systems and planning and directs a program in organization studies.

STEPHEN R. THOMAS received his undergraduate degree from Oberlin College. He taught at Westminster College, Smith College, and the Harvard School of Public Health while working toward a Ph.D. in government from the Graduate School of Arts and Sciences at Harvard University, which he received in 1980. Between 1980 and 1987, Dr. Thomas was Assistant Professor of Political Science and Environmental Policy in the

Department of Health Policy and Management, Harvard University School of Public Health. Dr. Thomas' interests, in addition to health policy, include political theory, environmental policy, and public management. He is the author of *Asking the Wrong Questions: Environmental Protection in the Carter Years*. Among his numerous consulting and service activities, Dr. Thomas was active in New England town government and worked with the federal Environmental Protection Agency to train its managers in environmental crisis management. In 1987, Dr. Thomas became Assistant Vice President for Program Policy at The Commonwealth Fund in New York, where he works on the development and management of the foundation's philanthropic agenda.

DAVID W. YOUNG is Professor of Accounting and Control in the School of Management at Boston University, and is affiliated with the School's Health Management and Public Management Programs. He is on the faculty for the Program for Chiefs of Clinical Service at Harvard University, and has consulted for such diverse organizations as the Ochsner Foundation, CIGNA Corporation, the Hospital Corporation of America, the Michigan Division of Insurance, the American Arbitration Association, the New York City Bureau of the Budget, and the Kuwait Ministry of Public Health. He is widely published in the health policy and management literature, and is the author of *Management Control in Nonprofit Organizations* (with Robert N. Anthony), *The Hospital Power Equilibrium: Physician Behavior and Cost Control* (with Richard B. Saltman), and *Financial Control in Health Care: A Managerial Perspective*. He received an M.A. in economics from the University of California at Los Angeles, a D.B.A. from Harvard University, and was a Milton Fund Fellow at Harvard Medical School.

LYNN B. JENKINS received her master's degree in education from Harvard University in 1988. Her master's studies have been concentrated in the area of writing research; recent work includes a series of case studies investigating the developmental histories of expert writers. Ms. Jenkins presently serves as a writing consultant to the Cambridge Arts Council, and as a writer and editor for the Publications Office at the Harvard Graduate School of Education. She previously worked as a Research Associate in the Program Evaluation Unit at the Massachusetts Mental Health Center in Boston, where her research activities included a cost-effectiveness analysis of psychiatric treatment alternatives, funded by the National Institute of Mental Health, and survey research on a leadership training program for state mental health directors.

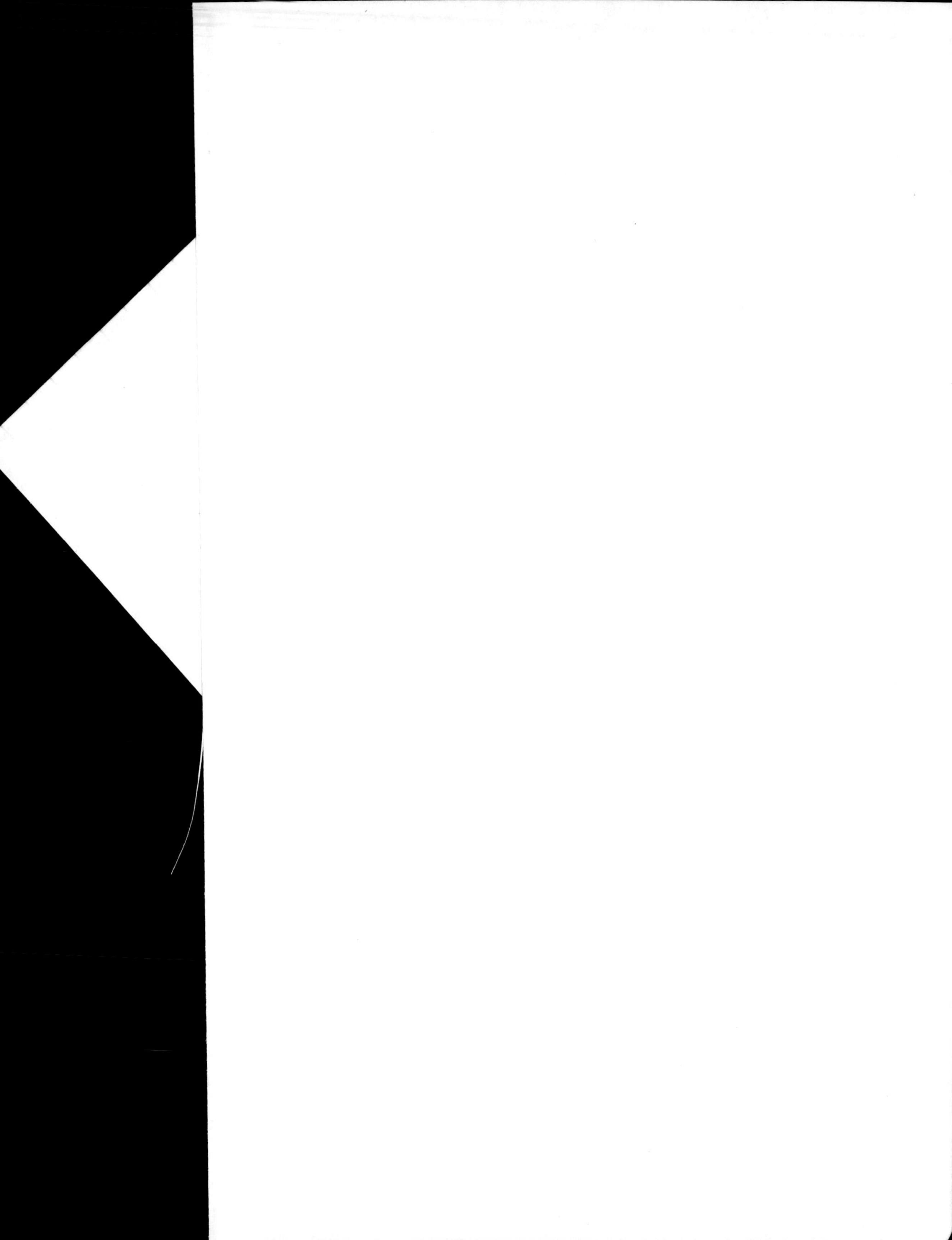

SEP 2 1989
DEC 14 1995
MAR 25 2000
HIGHSMITH 45-220